The Moral Work of Nursing
Asking and Living with the Questions

Hazel J. Magnussen

PROMONTORY
P R E S S

The Moral Work of Nursing:
Asking and Living with the Questions

Copyright © 2014 Hazel Magnussen
Promontory Press Inc.
Victoria, Canada
www.promontorypress.com

First Edition: May 2014

Library and Archives Canada Cataloguing in Publication

Magnussen, Hazel J., 1943-, author
    The moral work of nursing : asking and living with the questions / Hazel J. Magnussen. — First edition.

Includes bibliographical references.
Issued in print and electronic formats.
ISBN 978-1-927559-50-5 (pbk.).—ISBN 978-1-927559-51-2 (pdf)

    1. Nursing ethics. 2. Medical ethics. 3. Nursing—Canada.
4. Medical care—Canada. 5. Magnussen, Hazel J., 1943-. I. Title.

RT85.M34 2014   174.2   C2014-901146-6
                                       C2014-901147-4

Cover Design by SpicaBookDesign
Typeset in Constantia

Printed in India
0 9 8 7 6 5 4 3 2

TABLE OF CONTENTS

Dedicated to

**Nurses of the Past, Present and Future
who have done and continue to do
the Moral Work of Nursing**

WILDFLOWER

She's faced the hardest times you can imagine
And many times her eyes fought back the tears
And when her youthful world was about to fall in
Each time her slender shoulders
Bore the weight of all her fears
And a sorrow no one hears
Still rings in midnight silence in her ears

Let her cry, for she's a lady
Let her dream, for she's a child
Let the rain fall down upon her
She's a free and gentle flower
growing wild

And if by chance that I should hold her
Let me hold her for a time
But if allowed just one possession
I would pick her from the garden to be mine

Be careful how you touch her for she'll awaken
And sleep's the only freedom that she knows
And when you walk into her eyes you won't believe
The way she's always paying for a debt she never owes
And a silent wind still blows that only she can hear
And so she goes

Let her cry, for she's a lady
Let her dream, for she's a child
Let the rain fall down upon her
She's a free and gentle flower
growing wild

The song WILDFLOWER is based on this poem written in 1970
by David Richardson, a young policeman in Saanich, B.C.,
for his girlfriend who was a nurse at Royal Jubilee
Hospital. www.wildflowersong.com.

FOREWORD

It is my pleasure to have the opportunity to offer this foreword for Ms. Magnussen's unique and insightful book. Throughout it, she weaves a compelling narrative of her own history studying, practicing and living ethical practice in nursing and health care. Alongside Ms. Magnussen's personal historical narrative are her astute analytic commentaries on how nursing and health care have evolved to the present day. Her commentaries are effectively supported by her observations as well as related literature.

Ms. Magnussen writes this book from her standpoint as a retired expert in ethical practice in nursing and health care. She uses her personal narrative to encourage reflection on the part of her readers, explaining that "reflection nurtures curiosity, creativity and courage to ask questions and act ethically"(p. xv). Indeed, she models such reflections in the eleven chapters of her book—chapters which describe her initiation into nursing and her career foci and interests (Chapters One through Six), and move to her insightful observations about contemporary ethical challenges in nurses' workplaces (Chapter Seven through Ten). In fulfilling her reflective commitment, Ms. Magnussen closes her book in Chapter Eleven by discussing the meaning of spirituality and how spirituality and the events in her life and career have been intertwined.

The substance of Chapters Seven through Ten in

Ms. Magnussen's book is especially salient in today's era of increasingly constrained health care resources and increasingly stressed workplaces. For example, in Chapter Seven, Ms. Magnussen provides a comprehensive overview of moral distress in nursing practice, and she concludes Chapter Ten by providing strategies for addressing workplace bullying and restoring trust in health care workplaces. She links her analyses and recommendations to salient policies such as the Canadian Nurses Association (2012a) recent document, *A nursing call to action: The health of our nation, the future of our health care system.* Further, Ms. Magnussen's observation that "silence is part of nursing history and culture"(p. 69) is an important caution as our profession moves forward to strengthen our identity, our expertise, and our influence in health care and health policy.

I believe that Ms. Magnussen's book will be of interest to student nurses, nurses who wish to reflect on their own practice, nurse leaders at every level, and anyone studying ethics in nursing practice. Historians of nursing and health care will also appreciate Ms. Magnussen's unique experiences and vantage points.

Patricia Rodney

Patricia (Paddy) Rodney, RN, MSN, PhD
Associate Professor, University of British Columbia School of Nursing Faculty Associate, University of British Columbia Centre for Applied Ethics

PREFACE

When growing up on a farm in Alberta in the 1950's, I imagined making a difference in the world and after graduating from nursing school, I thrived in workplaces that welcomed my idealism. From a naive new graduate and novice manager, I grew with experience in a variety of clinical settings to become a seasoned professional. I was touched by those who entrusted me with their care and shaped by challenges along the way.

Over the years, I learned that the moral work of nursing can be difficult. After undertaking formal studies in health care ethics, I was surprised that some bioethicists did not consider nurses moral agents. Nursing was viewed as an extension of medicine and nurses often did not have a voice in moral decisions. Those in positions of power were reluctant to even acknowledge, let alone address, the power issues that contributed to demoralization within nursing.

Amid constant change, economic and political setbacks, nurses face daily challenges to provide safe, competent and ethical care in a system that may not take their concerns seriously. They are honoured to be part of critical events in people's lives; but when they dare to ask questions or advocate for improvements in health care services, the moral work of nursing comes with a cost. Nurses experience moral distress when they are unable to meet their professional obligations in a modern health care system often guided by economics and entrenched power structures.

Reflections on my own experience and other nurses' stories during the past fifty years provide deeper insights into the profession. Readers are invited to ponder the question: "Why is nurses' work, often invisible, frequently taken for granted, misunderstood and even discounted?" These reflections are intended to inform and increase readers' appreciation and understanding of the moral nature of nursing. Sometimes raising more questions than answers, they are meant to encourage critical thinking and inspire creative action. Support and psychological health and safety in the health care workplace are essential for all health professionals to do their work effectively.

As a retired nurse, my passion for nursing has not waned, but fuels my hope that the profession will flourish as nurses continue to make a difference in the lives of others.

Hazel J. (Schattschneider) Magnussen

ACKNOWLEDGEMENTS

Friends and colleagues, who reviewed and offered suggestions for the manuscript, validated and encouraged me to complete a project so close to my heart.

My husband, Lloyd, who provided moral and computer support throughout this undertaking.

Patricia (Paddy) Rodney, University of British Columbia School of Nursing Professor and author of this book's Foreword.

Anita Mozahn, Dean, Faculty of Nursing, University of Alberta, whose comment appears on the back cover.

Jane Burton, freelance editor, who reviewed numerous versions of the book manuscript during the past few years.

Carolyn Redl, colleague in the Canadian Federation of University Women's club, who provided an academic critique of a later version of the manuscript.

Ben Coles, Promontory Press, whose vision for publishing in the 21st century has made this book a reality.

INTRODUCTION

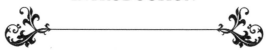

This book is the product of over forty years of first-hand experience, study, reflections on the meaning of nursing and its moral work. It includes an overview of nursing ethics and the effects of social and political developments on nursing during the past fifty years.

Connecting professional memories with news reports, ethics theory and related research, it is an example of reflective practice. Reflection integrates theory and practice, enables the practitioner to intuitively learn from experience, make connections with similar events and apply that learning to new situations (Mann, Gordon, & MacLeod, 2009; Ruth-Sahd, 2003). While requiring time and trust in colleagues or mentors when exploring new insights, reflection nurtures curiosity, creativity and courage to ask questions and act ethically.

The word *ethic* comes from the Greek word meaning "character." In its plural form, *ethics* refers to *moral philosophy* that concerns itself with "the principles of human duty and notions of the good. When applied to the characteristic spirit and prevalent tone of the sentiment of a people of a community, it is called *ethos*" (Benner, & Cook, 2011, p.1). Ethical reflection is essential in the moral work of nursing. David Seedhouse (2009), who believes that "work for health" is a moral endeavor, states in the preface of the third edition of his book, *Ethics: The Heart of Health Care*:

> The conceptually inadequate culture of conventional health care is hardly changed since I wrote the first edition of this book [1987]. The medical system continues to confuse clinical technique with health work; ethicists tell clinical students they must obey moral rules and principles if they want to be ethical; and countless opportunities to improve health go begging every day because most health professionals don't reflect deeply enough on the purpose to their work (p. v).

Rather than the traditional case study approach, this book uses narrative, as recommended by Brown and Rodney (2007), to facilitate ethical reflection. Since moral distress is linked to the organizational culture and socio-political context of situations, *The Moral Work of Nursing* focuses on personal narratives and broader issues affecting nurses' work. Questions for reflection and discussion are included at the end of each chapter.

The first chapter describes my initiation into the nursing profession as a student in the University of Alberta Hospital School of Nursing and after graduation, as a new graduate in an Alaska Native Hospital. Chapter Two summarizes my experience as the sole student in a new program to prepare nurses for work in the Canadian North, and concludes with updated information about midwifery and nurse practitioners in Canada. These chapters offer insight into the military traditions in nursing education, learning opportunities in northern nursing and elements of paternalism (or maternalism) in the health care culture of the time. Chapter Three describes a humanistic approach to nursing and an ethic that respects and encourages patients to participate in decisions affecting their care.

Chapter Four highlights how the growth of technology in the 1980's created new ethical issues in health care and how events surrounding infant deaths on two neonatal intensive care units impacted the nursing community. My subsequent study of the ethical implications of power in physician-nurse relationships is reviewed in Chapter Five. Chapter Six examines how reflection and dialogue help nurses clarify values, identify moral problems and take moral responsibility for their practice. The recurrent theme of moral distress experienced by nurses when that moral work is not supported by the health care system or specific workplaces is elaborated on in Chapter Seven.

Chapter Eight reviews the impact of health care reform and funding cut-backs in Canada during the 1990's, and draws attention to the invisibility of nursing, nursing workload and allocation of resources. The chapter concludes with discussion of the sustainability of the health care system and the Canadian Nurses Association's plan for nurses to lead the way in its transformation—shifting emphasis from acute care in hospitals to community care in primary care clinics.

Chapter Nine moves the focus from nursing practice to nurses' health. Discussing how the inability to act on one's values contributes to burn-out, I acknowledge my own mental health concerns resulting from workplace stress and conclude with suggestions for self-care. Chapter Ten elaborates on the significance of psychological health and safety in the workplace, and summarizes issues related to bullying—a phenomenon that includes or is also referred to as incivility, psychological harassment, mobbing, horizontal violence, relational aggression and disruptive behaviour. The chapter concludes with strategies for addressing workplace bullying and restoring trust in the health care workplace.

Nursing was, for me, a spiritual journey that I liken to walking the labyrinth. The ancient healing practice to integrate soul, body and mind is symbolic of the journey to the depths of one's being. Although the spiritual dimension of my story is implicit throughout the book, it is reviewed in the book's final chapter.

One
Initiation Into Nursing

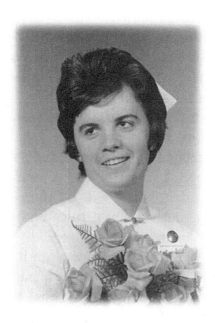

Dressed in a starchy white uniform and nurse's cap perched on her graying hair, exuding authority and warmth, she reached out to greet us as we walked through the door. "Welcome, I'm Miss Thomas, Director of the Nursing School. And you are..?"

Extending my hand, I replied, "I am Hazel Schattschneider."

"Hello, Miss Snaatsnider."

I did not have the nerve to correct her pronunciation of my name. In fact, the director continued to mispronounce my name until I corrected her during rehearsal for our graduation ceremony three years later. That may be surprising to those who know me now, but at that time and place, I was intimidated by the rule-oriented culture where one did not question, let alone correct authority.

On that first day, I simply turned to Mom and Dad standing beside me with my suitcases in hand. "I'd like you to meet my parents." They smiled proudly as Miss Thomas shook their hands.

Then, with the kind of efficiency and discipline about to become part of my new life, she announced, "I'll have someone show you to your room before your class meeting when I'll tell you more about your schedule. Residence staff will be there to give you information about residence rules and student services. Classes begin tomorrow."

I was an Alberta farm girl who, until my last year in high school, expected to become a teacher but then opted for nursing. The exploits of Nurse Cherry Ames, a fictional role model for girls growing up in the fifties, kindled my sense of adventure at an early age. Inspired by missionary nurses' accounts of life in foreign lands and encouragement from missionary relatives in Alaska, I felt called to become a nurse and **go North**! My teachers encouraged me to pursue more academic studies, apparently viewing nursing as a second rate choice. However, I stuck with my plan and wrote in my application letter (dated January 14, 1961):

> I have chosen nursing as my career because I like people and know that I will be able to give my best service to them through nursing. After getting my diploma in nursing, I would like to get my public health training and work among people in an underprivileged community. I look forward to facing the challenge that nursing presents.

In nursing school, the military metaphor, exemplified by words like training, dress codes, orders, duty, shifts and curfews set the tone for our lives. For example, we were expected to stand when physicians entered the nursing station. Just to be sure, I jumped up whenever any male approached the station area, even if he was a laboratory technician, medical student or orderly. We were to be obedient and loyal to physicians and others in authority. (Twenty years later, Winslow (1984) published an article entitled, "From Loyalty to Advocacy: A new metaphor for nursing.")

Some classmates were put off by the rules and expectations and moved on to other life and career choices while the rest of us learned to live and work within the system. Nursing was then considered a service and "calling." That became clear when, after a five month period of probation, we received our nursing caps and recited the Florence Nightingale Pledge to "pass our lives in purity and practice our profession faithfully." Serving as chief nurse in the Crimean War, Florence Nightingale elevated the stature of nurses by insisting on cleanliness and order. On her return to Britain, she opened the St. Thomas Hospital School of Nursing in 1860 and continued her work as a reformer, author and educator. In Canada, the first trained nurses were members of religious orders, such as the Grey Nuns who opened hospitals in Ottawa in 1845 and later in western and northern parts of the country.

Our role models were dedicated women who taught the art and science of nursing and measured our practice by the precision of our clinical skills and thoroughness of our observations and reports. I do not recall any discussion about morality and ethics in those early days. Apparently, anyone who chose to become a nurse was expected to be upright and moral. The ethic of virtue and values of caring, integrity and discipline were to guide our practice.

Days were filled with classes in anatomy and physiology, pharmacology, nursing fundamentals and clinical specialties of medicine, surgery, obstetrics, pediatrics, psychiatry, nursing arts practice labs, ward assignments and private study. While we were in class, a Nursing Reserve of women (who had nursed for at least five years before leaving the workforce to raise their children) filled in to ensure adequate coverage of patient care. During our three years of "training" at the University of Alberta Hospital, students were assigned responsibilities ordinarily given to Registered Nurses—at times, even placed in charge of nursing units. Our service, in effect, paid for our education, books, uniforms, room and board and a monthly stipend of $12.50 for toiletries and shoe polish.

Facing death for the first time

Recollection of my initiation into nursing takes me back to my first clinical assignment in nursing school. Awkwardly completing one step at a time as a nervous novice, I was more focused on the procedure than the patient. In a discussion with my instructor later that week, she told me that the elderly lady had died. Regrettably, I had not realized how sick the patient was, but the act of washing the feet of that woman near the end of her life was a fitting beginning to my nursing education. That first clinical experience set me on a path of learning the meaning of empathy.

Along with witnessing birth, coming face to face with death is one of the most profound experiences in nursing. During a posting in the Colonel Mewburn Pavilion[i] early in my second year of nursing school, I was reminded of the myth that "death comes in threes." A former army hospital, the Mewburn continued to care for male patients on open wards with attached rooms for those who were seriously ill. Working evening shift, my assignment included nursing a terminally ill man dying with cancer. I remember his emaciated body, the thud of the needle hitting his hip bone when I gave him injections for pain, and my uneasiness as I turned him and tried to keep him comfortable. When he died, the nurse in charge assisted and taught me how to prepare his body before taking him to the morgue.

On another shift, I was assigned to a cardiac patient on a Levophed intravenous drip for low blood pressure. Without the gadgets of late twentieth century medicine to regulate the administration of intravenous medications, my main responsibility was to monitor his vital signs and adjust the drip to ensure that the patient did not receive more than 40 mcgm of the medication per minute. I do not recall any other medical details, but remember the scariness of seeing my patient suddenly go into cardiac distress and die. As a novice, I did not have the knowledge or experience to anticipate these events. Calling a Code for the resuscitation team was not an option at that time.

I knew nothing about these men's personal stories nor do I recall any dealings with their family members. Already shaken by two successive deaths, and without any opportunity to debrief the experiences with a clinical instructor, I was unprepared for another death. The third death later that week was not a patient—rather, it was my own beloved grandfather. Grandpa had been diagnosed with leukemia and admitted to another unit in the Pavilion the day before. When I went to visit him before reporting for evening shift, I was surprised to find his bed empty. He had died earlier in the day. I must have been in shock when attending Grandpa's funeral—a day I was required to make up two years later in order to qualify for graduation.

I am amazed that, seemingly, death was treated in such a matter of fact way. We were "trained" to do procedures one step at a time, practicing them on each other and then on the wards with patients. Discussion of the emotional and spiritual needs of the patient and the patient's family was not part of the procedure. When it came to caring for the dying patient, we learned about physical care, a little about pain management and the procedure for caring for the patient's body after death. Since then, I have had the privilege of sitting with and caring for other dying patients—truly sacred moments.

As in these examples, the regimentation of my training prepared me to handle difficult situations sometimes on my own or with another student. Staff nurses on the unit and neighbouring units, supervisors or instructors were available when we called them. Often, this was for technical assistance as our main support came from classmates as we swapped tales back in residence after a difficult shift. Our personal and professional lives were regulated and monitored in residence, the classroom and on the hospital wards, but we did enjoy a wonderful camaraderie that left us a lifetime legacy of friendship and memories.

Meanwhile, professional nursing organizations were advocating for the removal of nursing education from hospitals dependent on nursing students for service. A Canadian study of nursing education for the Royal Commission on Health Services concluded in its 1964 report: "The education system for nurses should be organized and financed like other forms of professional education" (Wilson, 1977, p.110).[ii]

I had chosen the University Hospital for my basic nursing education expecting that it would be the first step to further learning. For those in my class already pursuing a degree in nursing, the three year diploma program was sandwiched between two years at university. A four year degree program was introduced in 1967. Returning to the University of Alberta to complete my Bachelor of Science degree in nursing in 1972, I welcomed the opportunity to broaden my education but nursing ethics was still not on the curriculum.

Trustworthiness: an essential ingredient in health care

So what were the moral dimensions of my early nursing education? Along with discipline and the work ethic, *trustworthiness* stands out as a virtue crucial in our work and interactions with others. Surely, the hospital counted on our trustworthiness to carry out our ward and patient care assignments often with little supervision. Yet it was seldom discussed, often taken for granted but still essential for safe, ethical health care. An experience during a surgical posting prior to graduation exemplifies its importance.

Narcotics are routinely locked in the narcotics cupboard and were counted at the end of each shift. The keys to the cupboard were carried by a registered nurse or student, who was responsible for recording the administration of narcotics on the narcotics record. One evening, after completing my first round of post-operative patient checks, I entered the nursing station. Seeing the ward clerk at the desk, I said, "Where is the nurse in charge?"

She replied, "She's gone for supper."

Surprised that the nurse had not checked in with me before leaving, I said, "But where are the narcotic keys?"

She replied, "I've got them. She always leaves them with me. Do you need them?"

Gasping at this breach in protocol, I approached her with an outstretched hand. "Yes, I'll take them. Thank you."

I recalled the incident several weeks after completing that posting, when I learned that police intercepted and arrested the ward clerk as she was leaving work with stolen drugs. I was stunned! I knew she had access to the narcotic keys but how did she get caught stealing drugs?

Apparently, the head nurse became suspicious when nurses consistently reported that analgesics were ineffective in relieving patients' pain. She contacted the authorities and surveillance cameras were set up in a building across the street to monitor activity around the narcotic cupboard through the hospital window. Evidently, the ward clerk had been withdrawing narcotics from vials in the cupboard and replacing the medication with saline solution. I was well aware that the ward clerk should not have access to the narcotic keys. Even then, one could not assume that everyone working in the system is trustworthy. But how can health professionals work together without trusting each other?

Along with 67 other graduates from the Class of September '64, I moved from the security of nurses' residence to follow my dreams. On the successful completion of our nursing exams, we were licensed by the Alberta Association of Registered Nurses to practice as Registered Nurses in Alberta. While employed on the renal medical unit at the University Hospital, I completed the paper work necessary for employment in Alaska.

North to Alaska and learning from experience

In January 1965, four months after graduation, I travelled north to Alaska to work as a staff nurse in the United States Public Health Service Native Hospital in Bethel, a town of about 1000 people 450 miles west of Anchorage. The 65 bed hospital served the native people of southwestern Alaska; Yupik Eskimos living along the Kuskokwim River that empties into the Bering Sea, and Athapascan Indians in more northerly villages along the Yukon River winding its way to the sea from the Yukon Mountains. At least once a day, village community health workers talked on radio telephone with a hospital doctor who gave directions for treatment and ordered transportation to hospital, at times with a nurse escort, for those requiring medical attention. My innocence and idealism were about to be tested.

I enjoyed new working relationships that were less formal than in nursing school, adapted quickly to the clinical demands and learned about the traditions and lives of the native people. However, I was shocked by the magnitude of the area's health problems. When the general ward of the hospital was full with medical patients and over-flowing with children, nurses were required to work extra shifts to provide the necessary care. Respiratory infections were common, but contaminated village water contributed to *E. coli*

(*Escherichia coli*) bacterial infections that were often deadly for the babies. The infant mortality rate in that area at the time was one of the highest in the world (118 per 1000 births).

Some memories linger with me. I recall the warm welcome by local people and hospital staff from other states in the United States of America, the laughter and delight of the children on the ward when they watched and listened to the toilet flush—a new experience since their homes were equipped with *honey buckets;* my surprise when serving meals with the eyes of fish heads looking up at me; somber trips to the morgue at the end of the children's wing with dead babies and adult drowning victims of boating accidents on the mighty Kuskokwim River; and the peacefulness when picking berries on the spongy, grassy tundra with its autumn hues enhanced by brilliant sunsets on the distant horizon.

One particular critical incident placed me in the middle of a moral dilemma for the first time. I was working on the medical and pediatric ward filled with adult medical patients and dehydrated infants with gastroenteritis on intravenous drips requiring frequent checks. As the nurse in charge on the ward that evening, I was responsible for medications, supervision of staff, processing and carrying out doctor's orders, monitoring and recording the status of thirty or more patients. The shift supervisor advised me that a woman with gastroenteritis was being transferred from the maternity ward. If she remained on the maternity unit, other mothers and their newborns could become infected. I appreciated the dilemma but how could we monitor the woman's labour, assist with her delivery and still adequately care for other patients? I protested but to no avail.

The patient in labour was placed in a room at the end of the hall, but before we had a chance to properly set it up, the baby was born. When I saw that the baby was not breathing, I called for help, "Get the doctor! Bring the suction machine and the oxygen!!"

The nurse from the other unit and other staff scrambled to bring the necessary equipment. The nursing supervisor rushed to help. The doctor dashed over from his residence near the hospital but it was too late—the baby was dead. I do not remember what we said to the mother or what she said to us. I expect we expressed our regret. The stoic mother, who might already have lost one or even more than one child, may not have said anything. She was probably in shock and wondering what had gone wrong. I remember my own outrage and protest, "This shouldn't have happened!"

Others tried to console me, "You did all you could— it's not your fault." Apparently, I was supposed to take this unfortunate incident in stride and move on. Other patients needed my attention. I do not know why the baby died nor if we could have saved the baby had we been prepared. I just wish we could have done better.

We did not discuss the incident in moral terms but it taught me that health care may require tough ethical choices. Leah Curtin and Josephine Flaherty

(1982) explain the difference between an ethical problem and ethical dilemma:

> Every problem is not an ethical problem and every ethical problem is not a dilemma. *A dilemma is a choice between equally undesirable alternatives.* If the choice is between what one *ought* to do and what one *wants* to do, the person has a problem for which there is an answer. If the choice is between the greater of two goods or the lesser of two evils, one still has only a problem and an answer can be found. In a true dilemma, however, any action taken will result in an unfavourable outcome and/or will constitute a breach to one's duty to another (p. 45).

In the incident involving the patient in labour, the choice was between having her deliver on the maternity ward and put other mothers and newborns at risk for *E. coli* infections or moving her off the ward and placing her and her baby at risk. Neither option was favourable; yet the nursing supervisor was forced to make a choice.

I learned that standards drilled into me in nursing school were not always realistic or possible to meet. Shaking my head when caring for two children in one crib, I'd exclaim, "if only my instructors could see me now." Cringing when a dedicated and reliable nursing aide lined up the kids with butts in the air to take their temperatures, I was amazed at their attentiveness, remaining still until they were told they could move.

My Alaskan nursing experience provided amazing opportunities to consolidate my skills as a new graduate in a setting where my work was valued by colleagues and patients. On completion of my two-year contract, I was ready to move on with confidence and knowledge that nursing does make a difference. Privately though, I questioned the limitations of hospital nursing. With little, if any, knowledge of their living situations, we treated our patients and sent them home. Social conditions, inadequate housing and sanitation were obviously affecting people's health. I wanted to know more about their families and communities, and especially, how to decrease or prevent the number of infant deaths. (When I returned for a visit four years later, the number of infant deaths had decreased significantly as a result of effective public health measures to ensure clean water supplies in the villages.)

I was touched by the spirit and people of Alaska but was ready to return to Canada. Public health nursing had been my ultimate career goal so when I read about the inauguration of an Outpost Nursing program at Dalhousie University in Halifax, Nova Scotia (Dickinson, 1966), I wrote for more information.

Questions for reflection and discussion

1. Is nursing a 'calling'/vocation, career or a job? How is it different from 50 years ago?
2. What would you have done if you had discovered that the narcotic keys had been given to the ward clerk?

3. Do you believe the people with whom you work are trustworthy? How do you know?
4. In your view, did the nursing supervisor in the Alaska hospital make the right choice? Describe an example from your life or practice when you had to make a choice that would result in two equally unfavourable outcomes.

Two
Breaking Ground For the Education of Nurse Practitioners

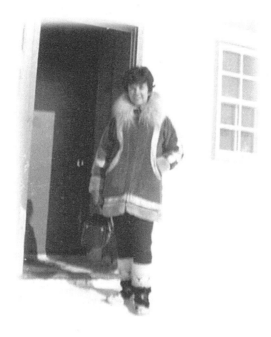

In September 1967, I boarded the eastbound train from Edmonton to Halifax, Nova Scotia, to become a student in a new program designed to prepare nurses for work in outposts in the Canadian North. By the end of the first year of the program with classes in clinical assessment, diagnostic and treatment skills in general medicine, pediatrics, midwifery and courses in abnormal psychology and public health nursing, three out of the five students left the program. Another left early in the second year. Some quit for personal reasons but, as a group, we believed the program requirements and schedule that extended past the regular academic term were unreasonable. I discussed our concerns with the director but apparently, the proposed time frame was not negotiable. Nevertheless, I resolved to stay to the end.

My second year began with a six month midwifery practicum in St. Anthony on the northern tip of Newfoundland. St. Anthony is the headquarters of the International Grenfell Association, a health service founded by Dr. Wilfred Grenfell on the Newfoundland and Labrador coast of eastern Canada in 1914. My internship included experience in the community and hospital where I monitored pregnant women through their pregnancies and labours, and assisted in the babies' deliveries. I was grateful for instruction and encouragement from mentors and the privilege granted by 38 mothers to deliver their babies. Midwifery provided the profound experience of being with women during their childbearing and delivery experiences and supporting them as they bonded with their new babies.

The second half of my one year internship was with Health and Welfare Canada in its Baffin Zone of the Northwest Territories.[iii] Without a plan or schedule for the practicum, as the lone student, my first assignment was working with physicians at the Frobisher

Bay Hospital. A pediatric resident supervised me in doing patient histories and examinations.

After a few weeks, I was sent to the nursing station in Igloolik, a settlement of about seven hundred people at the time. It is located on an island northwest of Frobisher in the Fox Basin on the east edge of Melville Peninsula. The two nurses there were both trained midwives and responsible for 24 hour health services in the community. Physicians in Frobisher Bay were available for consultation on radio telephone. The nursing station had clinic space, sleeping quarters for one or two patients and living quarters for staff. It was a difficult month living in close quarters with two other nurses who had little space or time to themselves. Since they were not sure what to do with me, I was assigned kitchen duties but also worked in the clinic. It was especially busy when the flu spread through the community. Three sick babies were admitted as inpatients in the Centre while we waited for suitable weather for an airplane to evacuate them to hospital. A new baby was delivered by one of the nurse-midwives in the nursing station during that month.

On my return to Frobisher Bay, I worked primarily at the Public Health Centre as a regular staff nurse in school and well-baby clinics. Along with the interpreter on staff, home visits were made to follow-up on people who had been exposed to or being treated for tuberculosis.

I returned to Halifax for Convocation in May, received diplomas in Public Health Nursing and

Outpost Nursing and was awarded the Outpost Nursing Prize. A Canadian Press story reported that the graduation of the first outpost nurse from Dalhousie University marked a significant milestone not only for the University's School of Nursing but for specialized nursing in Canada.[iv] I had already written two articles about the program (Schattschneider, 1969a, 1969b) and hoped that my completion of the program would make a difference for northern nursing in the future.

Since I was required to work until the end of June—the official end date of the course, I returned to Frobisher Bay after the convocation ceremony. When given the option of writing a research paper during those final weeks, I chose to examine patterns of communication between health and social service agencies, patients, and families when patients were sent to southern cities for medical treatment. I had noted that these patients and families were often separated and out of touch with each other for long periods of time.

In spite of the successful completion of the program and a couple of job offers, I knew I was not suited for work in an isolated outpost. I admired the commitment of northern nurses but was troubled by vestiges of colonialism in the system. I moved to Fort McMurray in northern Alberta, where my work as a municipal nurse included travel to outlying native communities. Eventually, I learned that health care is ideally a partnership among care recipients, families, communities and health professionals.

Progress in education and regulation of midwives and nurse practitioners

At the time of my midwifery practicum, many nurses working in northern nursing stations were mid-wives—often with training within the British system. Others may have taken the course in Advanced Practical Obstetrics offered at the Faculty of Nursing at the University of Alberta. That program was phased out in the 1980's and replaced in 1988 with a certificate in nurse midwifery in conjunction with the university's Master of Nursing program.

When circumstances and policies changed so that midwifery care was no longer available in northern nursing stations, expectant mothers were evacuated to the nearest community hospital for delivery. As a result, they were separated from their families for extended periods of time. When women, community leaders and health care providers saw the need for culturally appropriate midwifery services closer to home, birthing centres such as one in Rankin Inlet, Nunavut, were established. The National Aboriginal Council of Midwives (2013), established in 2008, now promotes reproductive health of Inuit, First Nations and Metis women and advocates for midwifery, education services and choice of birthplace for aboriginal people.

Educational preparation for midwifery practice is a four year baccalaureate program now available at seven Canadian universities, including an aboriginal midwifery program at the University College of the North in The Pas, Manitoba. In partnership with

Nunavut Arctic College and Laurentian University, Beverley O'Brien, registered midwife and nursing professor at the University of Alberta (2013) helped develop a midwifery program for Nunavut in the eastern Arctic. The course includes O'Brien's new book, *Birth on the Land: Memories of Inuit elders and traditional medicine,* describing Inuit birthing practices and traditions. These developments reflect a shift from a colonial approach to health care to one that involves and respects aboriginal people and their traditions.

Meanwhile, other women across Canada are also choosing midwives as their primary care givers for the full scope of their maternity care. Midwifery was first regulated in Ontario and Alberta in 1994. Currently, most provinces and territories (except for New Brunswick, Prince Edward Island, Newfoundland and Yukon) have licensed practicing midwives. Picard (2013) notes that the 900 midwives in Canada are underused and misused; and describes the disbanding of the New Brunswick midwifery licensing body by its government in 2013 as "a striking example of the reluctance in Canadian health care to do anything different no matter how untenable the status quo". He reports that childbirth is the No. 1 cause of hospital admission in Canada, even though pregnancy is not a disease and natural childbirth does not generally require medical intervention. Picard concludes that the expansion of midwifery services would be smart health policy that cuts costs.

The Canadian Association of Midwives (2013) letter

to the editor in response to Picard's article describes the status and merits of midwifery in *low risk maternity care*:

> Midwifery has been well documented in Canada and globally to provide safe and cost-effective care that reduces hospital admissions and re-admissions, reduces interventions, increases maternal satisfaction as well as optimal maternal and newborn health outcomes . . .
>
> Improving Canadian maternal and newborn health service delivery requires supporting midwives, family physicians, as well as perinatal nurses, rural physicians and nurse practitioners provide *low risk maternity care* as close to home as possible for all women in Canada.

Along with its focus on midwifery, the Dalhousie Outpost Nursing Program broke new ground in educating nurses for expanded practice as nurse practitioners in northern communities where physicians were not available. In 1971, McMaster and McGill universities also introduced nurse practitioner (NP) courses. The following year, other universities offered programs, in conjunction with Health and Welfare Canada, to upgrade the skills of nurses already working in northern settlements. Although physicians were available for radio/telephone consultation to northern nurses, their profession did not generally support the idea of nurse practitioners in southern communities where they might be perceived as doing physicians' work. In the North where there were fewer doctors, nurse practitioners were looked on favourably.

In the 1980's, according to Health Canada (2006), "NP initiatives ended due to a perceived oversupply of physicians and the lack of: a remuneration mechanism for NPs; applicable legislation; public awareness regarding the role of NPs; and support from both medicine and nursing" (p.1). However, with renewed interest in advanced nursing practice during the 1990's, Alberta became the first province to pass legislation for: "registered nurses providing 'extensive services' and enabled nurse practitioners to work in urban settings such as hospitals and community clinics" (Sinnema, 2011, p. A3). The following decade, the Canadian Nurse Practitioner Initiative (CNPI), funded by the Canadian government, established a framework for the integration of Nurse Practitioners into the health-care system (Canadian Nurses Association, 2009a).

Canada has more than 3000 nurse practitioners who are experienced registered nurses, educated at a master's level and certified by their provincial nursing regulatory authority for an expanded role in assessment and management of common health problems (Canadian Nurses Association, 2011). They do not replace or compete with physicians; rather, their work complements medical care and increases public access to health care. Some of Ontario's 1000 nurse practitioners head provincially funded primary health clinics to improve "quality of care through enhanced health promotion, disease prevention and chronic disease management, as well as improve care co-ordination and navigation of the health care system at the local level" (Ontario Ministry of Health & Long Term Care, 2013).

In spite of studies demonstrating cost savings when nurse practitioners are used to their full potential, they have been underutilized (Cheperdak & Sudbury, 2011; Picard, 2012). Nonetheless, that may change as Canadians demand increased access to health care. In May 2012, when only 70% of nurse practitioners licensed in British Columbia were employed, the BC government announced funding to create 190 nurse practitioner positions in the next three years. The Association representing BC nurse practitioners noted: "Nurse Practitioners are ideally positioned to provide care for BC's most vulnerable patients" (British Columbia Nurse Practitioner Association, 2012).

Dr. Michael Rachlis (2004) in *Prescription of Excellence: How innovation is saving Canada's health care system,* reports on an innovation in southwestern Saskatchewan when a physician worked with a nurse practitioner to provide health services after two other physicians left the area. The team expanded to three nurse practitioners and one physician on contract with the health region. As a result, the physician had more time to work with patients with complicated medical conditions. Rachlis (2004) states:

> Teamwork promotes equality among different health professionals. As a result, teamwork promotes efficiency. Our present system is very inefficient because specialists perform tasks that could be performed by

family doctors, family doctors do work that could be done by nurses and other health workers, and providers waste their time doing things that patients and families could do for themselves. Other sectors have moved away from hierarchical structures because they waste human resources at every level (p. 219).

Forty years after the graduation of the first nurse practitioners in Canada, their acceptance and full integration into the health care system is long overdue. By increasing public access to primary care, nurse practitioners, in collaboration with physicians, contribute to safe, ethical and competent health care for Canadians.

Questions for reflection and discussion

1. How has the history of colonialism affected health care for Inuit and First Nations people? How can nurses and other health professionals help break the cycle?

2. What birthing stories have you heard in your family, community or health care practice? Do you view pregnancy and childbirth as a natural phenomenon or as a medical condition? Are there ethical implications for either point of view?

3. Nurse Practitioners are now recognized by the nursing profession and legislation but the medical profession is apparently still reluctant to welcome them as part of the health care team. Name some strategies for addressing that issue.

Three
A Humanistic Approach to Nursing

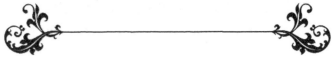

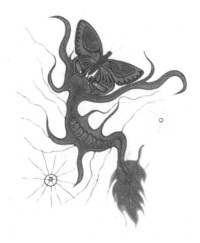

LIFE by Norman Knott

Although we believe that the essence of human actions lies
in the heart and soul found in them, actions are judged by the
difference they make in the world. Effective nursing practice
depends as much on the humanity of the nurse as it does on
the nurse's knowledge and technical skill
(Curtin and Flaherty, 1982, p. xv).

The above quote from a nursing ethics text is a fitting
beginning for reflection on a humanistic approach
to nursing—one guided by moral values such as

respect, dignity and choice. Human relationships are central to the practice of nursing and the nurse-patient relationship is its moral foundation (Yarling & McElmurry, 1986).

Throughout my career, I was privileged to practice in nursing roles as caregiver, coordinator, leader/manager, advocate, counselor and educator. Some likened me to a "butterfly" moving from one challenge to another, but few understood my metamorphosis as I struggled to break free from institutional restraints while hanging on to my moral values. A wide range of experiences expanded my horizons culturally, geographically and professionally and taught me the importance of seeing beyond myself in order to learn from others.

Much of my nursing work was in community, long term care and rehabilitation settings where the focus was not so much on treatment and cure but on care, support and health promotion. When medical and nursing care of the elderly and disabled expanded to include rehabilitation and social services, the multidisciplinary team evolved. Each discipline is challenged to be flexible and respectful of each other's expertise and contribution to the team. The Registered Nurses Association of Ontario in its 50th anniversary publication, *NURSE*, aptly describes Canadian health care in 1975:

> The health care system throughout history has fallen into distinct categories during its development. By necessity the beginning of care for the sick or the

afflicted rested in the hands of the immediate circle of family and friends; . . . [until] improved communications and transport created the possibility of organized care outside the home. The influence of the doctor and nurse grew with the dissemination of information. Hospitals grew in size as well as in prominence in the community and the mystery of medicine deepened into the application of its science and the attendant humanism has passed into the hands of a relatively few people . . .

. . . Eventually, society gave a sense of identity back to the sick and distressed. Today, care of all but the seriously ill patient is gradually returning to the home, with the support of a variety of health care professionals (Handbury, 1975, p.106).

Having embraced Joyce Travelbee's (1966) description of nursing as a human–to–human relationship that assists "an individual, family, or community to prevent or cope with the experience of illness and suffering, and if necessary, to find meaning in these experiences" (p.7), I believe the attendant *humanism* that accompanies the application of medical science is part of nursing.

I thrived in innovative positions, such as a pilot project funded by the Alberta government to learn whether attendance at a Day Hospital program would delay the institutionalization of elderly persons (Schattschneider, 1977). The Day Hospital integrated medical, nursing, rehabilitation services; but its social focus was especially beneficial for the seniors while their caregivers welcomed the respite. (Adult Day Centres now offer social and recreational programs that complement home care nursing and support services.)

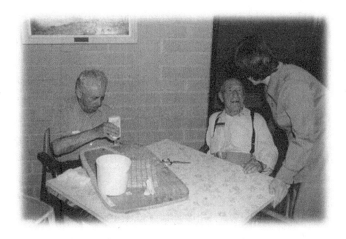

Another project was designed to improve psychosocial care of residents in nursing homes. A textbook edited by American nurse educator Irene Mortenson Burnside was a useful resource that, even now, offers timeless advice such as these words from one of its contributors (Herr, 1976):

> Nurses must be given the time, training and recognition for performing the essential psychosocial services the patients and their families require. For in the end, it is the responsibility of the *nursing profession to recognize that when nurses fail to fulfill their psychosocial treatment* obligations, patients and their families are apt to suffer iatrogenic consequences (p.44).[v]

Although progress was made in this regard, more recent organizational and funding models in long-term care facilities provide little time for psychosocial care. Staff become frustrated and experience moral distress when they recognize the consequences of lack of social interaction, activity and exercise for residents. [vi]

In the 1980's, nursing theory, a conceptualization of the nature of nursing, was especially popular in nursing education. Although I did not follow any particular theorist, I was hired as a clinical nurse specialist in an Ontario long term hospital because of my interest in ethics and humanistic approach to nursing. I was writing my master's thesis at the time. Gail Mitchell, another clinical nurse specialist, told me about a group of theorists who supported an approach consistent with my own. She was a student of Parse (1992) who described nursing as a human rather than natural science. Parse's theory of Human Becoming emphasizes that, rather than being fragmented into systems or parts, human beings are unified beings who, in interaction with their environment, are co-creators of their health. Using language such as *transcending* and *finding meaning,* Parse's theory reflects the spiritual nature of nurse-patient interactions.

Meanwhile, the nursing diagnosis movement, guided by the North American Nursing Diagnosis Association (NANDA), developed a system of nursing diagnosis. Ironically, while nursing was attempting to define its distinctive nature, it was also adopting a diagnostic approach that did not foster the personalized care expounded and valued by our profession.

Mitchell later co-authored an article elaborating on Parse's theory as an alternative to nursing diagnosis:

> Seeking creative ways of being with the patient, the nurse is present to the person's unfolding toward personal hopes and dreams . . . The patient, not the caregiver, is the primary decision maker on health. Instead of labeling people with standardized words and phrases focused on problems, the nurse talks with the person as the individual world of meaning, important relationships and hopes are described. The strictly sequenced steps of the nursing process are appropriate for problem solving in the physical sciences. They fail to reflect the complex dynamics of human interrelationships (Mitchell & Santopinto, 1988, p. 27).

Learning from clients

Assessment of risk and patient safety concerns is a responsibility that is frequently assigned to nursing. Actions taken by health professionals to protect patients' safety are balanced with patients' needs for independence and right to make choices about their care and living situations. Legal language of patient rights is commonly used in debates regarding life and death situations while personal choices regarding matters, such as living arrangements, may raise moral questions. The answers are not always clear, but even then, health professionals may want to provide solutions. One woman stands out among my many teachers.

Living independently with the help of mobility

aids, she asked the physiotherapist and me for assistance in purchasing a specialty bed. At the specialty bed store, she told the salesperson, "I'm shopping for a bed with controls so that I can adjust the height and the head of the bed. I'm sure that if I can elevate the head of the bed myself, I will be able to get myself up and into my wheelchair."

The salesperson replied, "Let me show you one of our models and you can try it yourself to see how it works for you."

The client tested out the bed but when I noted her difficulty in transferring from bed to chair, I said in a patronizing tone, "If this doesn't work for you, we could arrange for home care staff to come in to help you get up every morning."

She responded indignantly, "How can you say that? Do you know what it's like to depend on someone else to do your personal care? I know that with the right set-up, this can work."

I added to the harm already done with a comment about having to accept her situation. Needless to say, the interaction came to an uncomfortable end. She persisted in her quest to find what she needed to maintain her independence.

When we met again two years later, the woman congratulated me on my interview on a fund-raising telethon for the Muscular Dystrophy Association. "You've changed. You showed respect when you spoke of the need for support for persons with disability—a welcome difference from the 'feel sorry pitch' that has been so common at telethons."

I recalled that encounter when studying Benner's research to identify competencies of intuitive expert nurses. One such competency is the coaching function that makes aspects of illness more accessible. Benner (1984) reports:

> Illness, pain, disfigurement, death and even birth are by and large culturally avoided and uncharted experiences ... Experience in addition to formal educational preparation is required for the development of this competency ... A deep understanding of the situation is required, and often the ways of being and coping are transmitted without words but by demonstrations, attitudes and reactions (p.89-90).

According to Benner (1984), the *helping role* includes:

> ... creating a climate for and establishing a commitment to healing ... presencing, being with a patient; maximizing the patient's participation and control in his or her own recovery ... providing emotional and informational support of patients' families (p.50).

For people with chronic or debilitating illness, *recovery* means successful management of their conditions. As health care professionals let go of control, power and vulnerability are shared with the patient/client. This is the power of caring.

Even in today's health care environment that places more emphasis on science and high-tech skills than health care relationships, the therapeutic value of the nurse-patient relationship remains constant. Respectful treatment of patients/clients as fellow human beings is a central component of the moral work of nursing.

Questions for reflection/discussion

1. Do you agree with the nurse ethicists' statement about effective nursing practice quoted at the beginning of the chapter?
2. What have you learned from patients/clients about nursing?
3. Describe your own practice. Does it focus more on technical skills, scientific knowledge or human relationships? How do you integrate these dimensions of your work?

Four
Growth of Technology Creates New Moral Issues

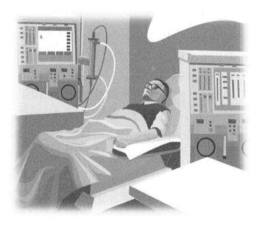

Advances in technology in the 1980's created new possibilities, expectations and moral issues. That became apparent to me while working in a clinic for people with neuromuscular disorders, characterized by progressive weakening of muscles, loss of mobility and in some cases, communication and respiratory function.

Innovative mechanical and electronic devices improve disabled persons' mobility, ability to communicate and control the environment. Meanwhile, the option of ventilator support when the respiratory system fails creates moral problems for clients and caregivers. Some choose that option and maintain a meaningful life. Nevertheless, one person with amyotrophic lateral sclerosis (ALS), an ultimately terminal condition, made it clear to me that she did not want extraordinary measures to prolong her life. When she was admitted to hospital with respiratory complications, I ensured that the physicians were aware of her wishes and she was allowed to die with dignity without invasive treatments.

Situations like this motivated me to learn more about palliative care, an alternative to life-saving measures when death is imminent. Hubert Doucet (1984), a Roman Catholic priest who taught health care ethics at St. Paul's University in Ottawa, describes *palliative care* as an ethical option:

> Palliative care, the purpose of which is to enable people to live out the last part of their lives with meaning and grace, ... makes us aware of the most fundamental aspect of ethics, and more. The art to dying, as embraced by palliative care, somehow leads us to go beyond such care to better appreciate its meaning (p.17).

Palliative care focuses on comfort measures and is not the same as *euthanasia,* which is the relief of a person's suffering by intentionally ending his/her life.

An incident in the neonatal intensive care unit in the hospital where I was employed drew attention to legal and ethical issues about *euthanasia* and premature infants. An audit of neonatal deaths noted that an infant had died forty minutes after receiving 15 mg of morphine (fifty times the normal infant dose). By law, the death should have been reported to the Office of Medical Examiners.

An investigation and subsequent public inquiry in 1983 revealed the facts of the case, which were summarized by journalist Sarah Growe (1991). The infant, delivered by emergency caesarean section due to pre-birth complications, was classified as a stillbirth but was revived after eight minutes of resuscitation. She was placed on a respirator and given intravenous fluids with orders for comfort measures and medications to prevent convulsions. A physician in attendance at the delivery later testified at the inquiry that the infant was not expected to live. Three and a half hours later when an electroencephalogram indicated that there was no brain activity, the baby's parents agreed to the removal of life support. When the baby's breathing and convulsions got worse, her nurse requested a medication order from the physician on duty to relieve the infant's distress. When she saw that the dosage ordered was excessive, she consulted with her supervisor who in turn checked with the physician. The medication was administered by the nurse with her supervisor present. She later testified in court that she knew the order was an overdose but wanted to relieve the baby's suffering.

The judge in the inquiry noted the autopsy did not establish that the "excessive and inappropriate" morphine dose caused the infant's death but added:

'The nurses wanted relief for the baby, her mother and grandmother. (The doctor) succumbed to 'additional requests by the nurses, and for some inexplicable reason, (the nurse), despite her experience, administered the drug in the dosage ordered by the doctor.' . . .

'Nurses have a duty to question a prescribed treatment.' But he (the judge) also spoke of the emotional tie nurses have for patients in their role as 'surrogate mothers' and recommended 'a continuing education psychological counseling program for nurses to assist them in overcoming this emotional tie. I wouldn't want them to get rid of it, just assist them in coping with it' (Growe, 1991, p.116-117).

Was the judge suggesting that the predicament arose because one nurse cared too much?

At a disciplinary hearing of the Alberta Association of Registered Nurses (AARN), the nurse who administered the medication and her supervisor were temporarily suspended from practicing nursing and called to testify at subsequent hearings. The Alberta College of Physicians and Surgeons suspended the license of the prescribing physician who had already left the country.

The Staff Nurses Association at the hospital kept members informed regarding the developments in the case. No matter what position any one of us took on the situation, we were all reminded of our vulnerability as nurses. I will never forget the president's words, "There but for the grace of God go I."

The harsh treatment of nurses after the unexplained deaths of infants at the Hospital for Sick Children in Toronto in 1981 was still fresh in our memories. Nurse Susan Nelles had been charged but later acquitted of the murder of four infants. Throughout the Grange Inquiry in early 1983 regarding the deaths, nurses were treated as suspects and their credibility undermined. Meanwhile, physicians were not challenged but used as expert witnesses. The subsequent report by the Registered Nurses Association of Ontario was dedicated to all nurses stating:

> To those who sound the alarm and are heard; to those who have questions they cannot voice and those who are held accountable for systems which are not theirs. It is dedicated too, to those nurses who work to be effective agents of change. *(Registered Nurses Association of Ontario RNAO, 1987)*

During the Taschuk Inquiry in Alberta held the same year as the Grange Inquiry in Ontario, nurses were wondering how nursing could again be under such severe scrutiny. We needed to know more about the situation. Could the crisis in the Alberta hospital have been prevented? Was any thought given to the potential aftermath of such extraordinary measures after delivery? Why would a stillborn even be resuscitated? Was this stretching the physician's duty to preserve life—life that, in this case, was apparently not evident in an infant who had asphyxiated during birth?

Growe (1991) quotes one doctor's testimony at the inquiry: "I do not embark on heroics if I have grave reservations, but with asphyxia, it's hard to tell. However, I guess you don't know until you try. You are committed to trying, and the problem is once you are committed to trying that means a flat-out, all-out effort" (p. 114).

Once the *medical machine* started, it was apparently not willing or able to stop after four minutes, even though brain cells begin to die without oxygen for four or more minutes. The status of the baby, already with significant brain injury, had not changed. I use the term, *medical machine,* to describe the depersonalization and mechanization of health care that is driven by an apparent need to save life at all costs regardless of the patient's wishes or prognosis.

Resuscitation efforts continued for another four minutes when the baby was revived with an Apgar rating of 1 out of 10 and "severe cerebral dysfunction." The nurses were then left to care for the dying child and grieving family. The disturbing dilemma might have been avoided if the medical machine had stopped earlier when it could see it was losing the battle. Were the actions that created a second crisis considered reasonable and ethical?

Resuscitation of tiny premature infants and frail, dying elderly patients had already become common practice often causing unnecessary trauma and prolonging death rather than preserving life. Off the record, some admitted that such scenarios provided opportunities for practicing resuscitation techniques.

Nurses who worked in critical care areas were known to say that they would have DNR (Do Not Resuscitate) tattooed on their chests in order to ensure they didn't meet a similar fate. As "health care consumers" were becoming more involved in decisions regarding their care, policies were developed for recording their wishes regarding resuscitation and other extra-ordinary measures to prolong life (or death).

Informed consent for surgery or other invasive procedures is standard practice. The roles of nurses as advocates and educators are essential to ensure that patients have adequate information in order to make informed decisions about their care. However, such decisions are easier when the use of technology is balanced with an alternative approach that, rather than treating death as the enemy, accepts death as part of life and allows people to die with dignity (Schattschneider, 1993).

Legislation now offers a defense against unsolicited treatment by enabling persons to provide advance directives for personal health care decisions. Although not applicable in the case of a newborn in distress, a legal document expressing one's wishes regarding end of life care can be useful for family and the health care team.[vii] However, dilemmas may arise when family members have different interpretations of their loved one's wishes; or when they refuse the discontinuation of life support even when its continuation is deemed futile by the physician.[viii]

Although technology provides new diagnostic methods and life-saving treatments, it creates new dilemmas and difficult choices for patients and health professionals. Health care ethics require continual examination and reflection on the use of technology and attention to what is in the best interest of the patient and the common good.

Questions for reflection and discussion

1. Do you agree with Hubert Doucet's description of palliative care? What does palliative care mean to you?

2. What would you have done if you were the nurse receiving the morphine order in NICU? If you worked on that Unit, how would you have supported the suspended nurses?

3. As a member of the general public, what is your response when cases such as these are reported in the news media?

4. Give an example of how you have advocated for patients and ensured that they and health care decision makers had enough information to make informed choices.

Five
Power in Physician-Nurse Relationships

Caring for and supporting patients coping with illness, disability and loss—the essence of nursing—was indeed a privilege, but the politics in the health care workplace made the work more difficult. The treatment of nurses in two high profile cases referred to in the previous chapter was especially troubling. All too often, nurse–patient relationships and nurses' knowledge of patient and family concerns were simply ignored. Viewing these as moral issues and looking for ways to address the resulting demoralization within the profession, I began taking courses in philosophy and bioethics.

When St. Stephen's Theological College on the University of Alberta campus established a Master's Degree program enabling lay people to integrate theology with their professional disciplines, I seized the opportunity to consolidate my studies in health care ethics. That choice gave me a chance to examine nursing and health care from the outside and recognize issues I may never have recognized from within the system.

I wrote my thesis on how power in physician-nurse-patient relationships affects nurses' work and participation in ethical decision-making. It reviewed the study of powers and principalities by New Testament theologian Walter Wink (1984, 1986) and writings by feminist theologians (such as Harrison, 1981 & Russell, 1974) raising consciousness and offering alternatives to patriarchal systems. To better understand health care ethics from a power perspective, those reviews were applied to exemplars of nursing practice from Patricia Benner's (1984) research on excellence and power in clinical nursing practice. My program included courses, projects and a clinical practicum in the intensive care unit in an Ontario hospital under the supervision of its chaplain.

I began asking the moral questions. Should the patient have a right to refuse extra-ordinary treatment measures? How should that choice be documented and honoured in accordance with the law? Should life-saving measures be undertaken simply because they are available? I had encountered these questions in my nursing practice, so was surprised to discover that some bioethicists at that time did not consider nurses to be moral agents.

For example, Veatch (1981) argued "that although 'nursing ethics' may deal with the unique moral problems faced by nurses, it is a limited term referring to a field that is a subcategory of medical ethics" (p.17). I was troubled by Veatch's restrictive view of the moral work of nursing, but was spurred on by the observations of Freedman (1981), a Montreal bioethicist, who noted:

> Nurses are the missing middle term in decisions of
> medical ethics, which tends to concentrate upon phy-
> sician-patient interactions, to the relative exclusion
> of patient-nurse or nurse-physician relationships.
> The significance of these latter relationships for eth-
> ical understanding cannot be denied particularly for
> the analysis of physicians and authority, yet they suf-
> fer from a paucity of ethical discussion (p.175).

Apparently, when developing a rational, principled
approach to health care ethics, leaders in the bioethics movement at the Kennedy Institute of Ethics at
Georgetown University in Washington, DC, focused
on medicine. Of course, the knowledge and skill of
the medical profession is critical in health care but
medical care includes collaboration with other health
care professionals.

Health care is a multi-disciplinary enterprise
that entails human encounters grounded in mutual
trust and respect. Patients and their families count
on health professionals to be competent and trustworthy. When all parties receive and pass on accu-
rate information, errors and tragic outcomes are less
likely to occur. While nurses rely on physicians to
be available to exchange vital information and write
and clarify orders, they are still held accountable
for their own actions. Physicians are most often the
entry point or gatekeepers to health care but nurses,
social workers, therapists and technicians are also
vital players. Those on the front lines, especially registered nurses and family physicians, are frequently

in the best position to listen, observe and advocate for patient needs and wishes.

If nurses' work and ability to identify moral issues and make ethical decisions are not recognized and valued, no wonder nurses become demoralized and distressed. Michael Yeo, Patricia Rodney, Pamela Khan and Anne Moorhouse (2010 a) describe the nature of moral autonomy and the development of moral agency:

> Through our actions or passivity, through words and silence, we can influence matters for good or ill. Becoming a more fully autonomous moral agent means accepting responsibility and being accountable for what we do or fail to do. It involves a continuing passage from a state of subjecting ourselves, with unquestioning loyalty or conformity, to the moral authority of others to a state of asserting authorship of our own moral lives (p. 350).

After completing my master's degree, I continued writing and shared my new understanding of ethics from a power perspective with nursing colleagues and friends who had similar concerns. I had learned that, in addition to power structures, organizations are guided by an inner ethos that sets the tone for interactions. Since these were radical insights for many in the establishment, this was "underground work." Yet hoping for opportunities to collaborate, I naively gave a copy of my thesis (Schattschneider, 1988) to a physician who had gained recognition as a local expert in medical ethics. He wrote a detailed critique that I shared with Walter Wink whose work I had used in my analysis of power in health care relationships. Wink (1993) later wrote about the physician's appraisal:

> In her Master's thesis, "Physician-Nurse-Patient Relationships: A nursing Perspective", Hazel Schattschneider employs an understanding of the Powers to analyze the role of nurses in Canadian hospitals . . .
> This milieu, which many nurses are trying to change toward a more collegial, interactive, relational set of power arrangements, is typically experienced as a system of "power over" rather than power sharing . . .
> This imbalance in power, which exists despite common knowledge that nurses are central to the healing process and are healers in their own right, has created an unhealthy corporate spirit or "angel" in hospitals that desperately requires transformation . . . .
> Critical to her argument is the assertion that it is not the personnel as such that create the problem, but the spirituality of the system that binds people into typified roles and responses . . .
> A medical doctor reviewing her thesis . . . will not concede that it has any relevance. He had never . . . recognized that the system over which he helps preside has an "angel" and now, having been apprised of its existence denies that nurses actually experience the patriarchal power system of the hospital as dehumanizing, demeaning and demonic, even after reading an entire thesis full of examples (p. 22-24).

Despite this physician's dismissal of my work, others such as the editors *of Humane Medicine* recognized its merits and published my article summarizing its conclusions (Schattschneider, 1990).

Shared moral work

Physician-nurse relationships are addressed by Janet Storch and Nuala Kenny (2007) in their discussion of shared moral work in health care:

> Together, nurses and doctors need to strive towards a better understanding of the enduring moral nature of a health care encounter from patients' perspective ... What we are missing is recognition of the essential and necessary interdependence and complementarity of the expertise of each profession and the need for a collaboration of commitment to the moral work of health care (p. 484).

They recommend that health professionals think of themselves as *workers* and consider their practice *moral work*. A *worker*, rather than *professional*, perspective focuses on the relational and organizational context of the work.

Even with the professional power imbalance between medicine and nursing, many physicians and nurses work together in the best interests of their patients. For example, early in my career, I shared moral work with physicians in Alaska as we cared for so many ill and dying babies. In mid-career, collaboration with the clinic medical director and physiotherapist in providing support for persons living with neuromuscular disorders was clearly moral work. Nurses in a northern Alberta hospital, in a tribute to a physician after his death, described their working relationship as partners in managing and sharing the burden of difficult clinical and moral situations:

> 'We affectionately remember Dr. Snider as a gentle spirit approachable by all. As colleagues, we felt supported, our professional judgment accepted and encouraged. With Dr. Snider, we enjoyed a comradery; we could tease, laugh and cry together. We could deal with acute cardiac situations, labor and delivery, psychological crisis, pediatric events and perform minor surgeries with competence … Being a rural physician, he was at the services of the community even when off duty and was a ready consultant to the neighboring nurse practitioner' (Magnussen, 2006, p.172).

Consciousness of moral work shared by physicians and nurses promotes mutual respect, addresses power imbalances, opens dialogue, welcomes questions and ultimately, improves patient care. The following chapter discusses the importance of reflection on practice and asking questions in nursing's moral work.

Questions for reflection and discussion

1. Who do you think holds the power in the health care system as a whole? Who holds the power in day to day health care decisions? Is there a need to address power imbalances?

2. Do you believe that nurses are moral agents? If so, how do they/you exercise that agency?

3. How do physician-nurse relationships differ when the focus is on shared work rather than professional status?

Six
Asking and Living with the Moral Questions

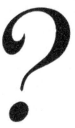

It costs so much to be a full human being that there are very few
who have the enlightenment or the courage to pay the price . . .
One has to abandon altogether the search for security, and reach
out to the risk of living with both arms.
One has to embrace the world like a lover.
One has to accept pain as a condition of existence.
One has to court doubt and darkness as the cost of knowing.
One needs a will stubborn in conflict, but apt always to total
acceptance of every consequence of living and dying.
(West, 2003, p.200-201)

Moral work begins with reflection on clinical practice, asking questions and recognizing ethical issues.
Answers to the questions may be ambiguous and res-
olution of the issues complicated, but we cannot avoid

the complexity and uncertainty that are part of professional life (Quinn & Smith, 1987). The ability to ask and live with the moral questions is essential for the work and wellbeing of nurses.

During a clinical ethics practicum in a hospital known for its research and surgical innovations, I asked a nurse if she ever questioned the ethics of the experimentation and its implications for patients. Without hesitation, she replied, "No, I don't think about it. If I asked such questions, I wouldn't be able to work here. I might be considered incompetent."

Does the nurse's response mean that in order to survive in the system, nurses should not ask questions? Are health care professionals being desensitized to moral issues and forfeiting their moral agency? When service cut-backs and organizational changes driven by economics compromise care, who will have the courage to speak up? And who will listen? Those who take the risk could lose their jobs.

In her review of the crisis in Canadian nursing, Growe (1991) documented an example of such a situation. In 1977, staff shortages prompted nurses at the Vancouver General hospital to go public with their concerns. They documented evidence of 60 incidents of unsafe patient care for the Registered Nurses Association of British Columbia (RNABC), their bargaining agent, but the nurses received no reply after the information was submitted to hospital administration. Instead, a nurse leader who supported her staff was forced to resign. Bonnie Lantz recalled that experience when elected as president of RNABC (2001) years later.

It was not accepted practice 23 years ago for nurse administrators to advocate for changes in a hospital system and I was fired for doing so. But my firing brought a group of nurses together who said, 'this is not right' and nursing made a powerful statement that we do have the right to identify issues that prevent us from providing safe care, and we need to be listened to (p. 13).

This scenario demonstrates that when nurses practice their moral agency, they can influence patient care and health care policy but may pay a price for their actions.

Ethical reflection and dialogue help nurses clarify values, identify moral problems and like the Vancouver nurses, take moral responsibility for their practice. Hardingham (2004) points out that rather than addressing moral concerns alone, nurses need to gather as moral communities in educational settings, workplaces and nursing organizations to reflect, encourage one another and strategize for change.

A Swedish study of 14 senior nursing students, who had learned to reflect and tell stories from their practice earlier in their education, described moral responsibility as "a relational way of being, which involved guidance by one's inner compass composed of ideals, values and knowledge that translate into a striving to do good" (Lindh, Severinsson, & Berg, 2007, p. 129).

A McGill University study (Beagan & Ells, 2007) interviewed 20 nurses to identify their values and the barriers to acting on those values in the workplace.

Values that mattered to these nurses were: *helping others, caring and compassion, making a difference, patient-centredness, patient advocacy, integrity, holistic care* and *sharing knowledge for patient empowerment.* When unable to act on their values, some described the "emotional toll" of burnout and detachment. They identified power relationships, workplace structures and the system's priorities as challenges to ethical practice.

In a three year project, "Leadership for Ethical Policy and Practice," a group of British Columbia nurse researchers (Storch, Rodney, Pauly, Fulton, Stevenson, Newton & Makaroff, 2009) worked with managers and other health care team members to examine nursing problems from an ethical perspective. Participants gained new insights and developed strategies to improve the ethical climate in the workplace. Managers' involvement and support for the goals of the project were essential for its success.

Workplace culture

Workplace culture, a primary influence on health care relationships, ultimately affects the moral work of health care professionals. Sociologist Arthur Frank (2005) used examples, mainly from medicine, to argue that health institutions ought to be places of hospitality and generosity that encourage dialogue. He uses the term:

> *Artificial person,* revived by philosopher Elizabeth Wolgast to describe how professional corporate

organizations generate dilemmas of moral responsibility . . . Artificial persons have administrative
utility because they act not on their own authority
but to implement an authority that resides elsewhere
(p. 126-127).

Frank notes that in such an environment, generosity in a moral relationship is transformed into an
administrative problem.

So how does the culture of the workplace affect
workers' generosity, ability to make moral choices
and provide safe, ethical care? Each institution has
a distinctive ethos reflecting its implicit moral code.
Symbols and rituals, such as assessment tools, meeting schedules and agendas and formal and informal
power structures are indicators of what drives the system. Mission statements posted in the workplace may
reflect an aspired goal that has not yet been achieved
as old mindsets and structures still guide much of the
practice.

The ideal work setting fosters respect for clients,
workers and visitors and is naturally open to new ideas,
feedback and self-examination in order to improve
practices. Collaboration is the norm. Employees are
encouraged to care, practice self-discipline and respect
clients and one another no matter what their background or position in life. Employers validate their
employees' work efforts, take measures to provide
healthy and safe workplaces and support ethical practice. Such settings are places of hospitality and generosity where guests/clients feel safe and welcome.

On the other hand, organizations that promote attitudes of power and control are more concerned with enforcing the rules and protecting the status quo than the well-being of their clients and workers. Employees are expected to act as *artificial persons* within set limits and regulations. Workplaces with a "fortress mentality" create suspicion of others outside that establishment. Competition is the norm. In a climate resistant to change, workers and clients become hesitant to ask questions or express opinions.

Some work settings have elements of both examples but the differences are recognizable to the shrewd observer. Certain organizations may be driven by ethnocentrism that assumes all people are the same, so inadvertently condone discrimination against those who are different. Again, an astute observer recognizes when such a cultural bias is present, even in the discipline of health care ethics.

Moral and cultural sensitivity

At a conference attended by bioethicists from across North America in 1989, discussions reflected the priorities and values of the cultural group (i.e. mostly urban, white, middle or upper class, well-educated academics) represented at the conference. I had just returned from the Canadian Arctic where Inuit mothers, who wanted to give birth closer to home, were asking for birthing centers in their home communities. I shared that example to draw attention to the cultural bias built into a particular discussion about fetal technology that ignored the more basic concerns of childbearing. Members of the group acknowledged the foregone conclusions of mainstream bioethics but, to my knowledge, the gist of that discussion was never recorded in the conference proceedings.

Obviously, others were asking similar questions since six years later, a new textbook, *Health Care Ethics in Canada* (Baylis, Downie, Freedman, Hoffmaster & Sherwin, 1995) was released. Describing changes in health care ethics in the earlier three decades, the preface states:

> For a long time, the role of culture in health care was invisible. Now, the profound ways in which culture affects the delivery of health care and the nature of health care ethics are being appreciated ... the contexts in which ethical issues arise always are important in shaping how those issues are perceived and resolved (p. v-vi).

That same year, I presented a paper reviewing research and reflections on Moral and Cultural Sensitivity in Bioethics at the annual conference of the Canadian Bioethics Society. It referred to the work of Madeline Leininger (1990) who pointed out that culture is the missing link in understanding the moral aspect of human care. In addition, Annette Brown's (1993) description of respect as a nursing ethic that "acknowledges the dignity, inherent worth and uniqueness of humans and their potential for self-determination" (p. 212) considered the cultural context. I also reviewed two anthropology studies (O'Neil, 1989;

Kaufert & O'Neil, 1990) of medical encounters with native clients. Analysis of the case studies revealed that the historical and political influences of a "colonial" system of native health care apparently contributed to insensitivity to culture and power imbalances in these clinical interactions.

According to Lawrence Blum (1991), *moral perception,* the ability to ferret out moral features of situations, involves moral and psychological notions such as salience, empathy and self-reflection. Moral sensitivity, perception or discernment considers the historical, political and cultural context in which a moral situation arises. When able to recognize their own personal, professional and cultural values and assumptions, health professionals can be more open to cultural diversity and sensitive to moral situations.

Psychologist James Rest (1982) identifies *sensitivity,* the ability to discern and identify moral problems, as the first of four components of ethical practice. The other three are *reasoning,* the capacity to ask questions and reflect on the issues; *commitment,* caring enough to make the moral choice even when there is a cost; and *action,* the interpersonal skills and ego strength to go forward in spite of adversity. Obviously, this work requires courage and determination.

Reflection and dialogue are necessary to identify moral issues and recognize how workplace relationships and culture can either impede or support ethical practice. The potential consequences of questioning unethical practices are discussed in the following chapter.

Questions for reflection and discussion

1. Name examples when you, other nurses or health professionals took a stand on issues affecting health care.

2. How much time do you take for self-reflection? What values are most important to you and how do they affect your practice? What are the barriers that stand in the way of acting on your values?

3. Have you encountered any "artificial persons" in your work or community? Have you ever been in a moral predicament that you were unable to resolve and dismissed as someone else's problem? How did you feel?

4. How do we acquire moral sensitivity? Is it possible that work in health care might desensitize workers to moral issues?

Seven
Moral Distress in Nursing

The cost of the moral work of nursing, such as losing one's job after speaking up for patient safety, has been alluded to in previous chapters. This chapter focuses on nurses' distress when systemic or other constraints make it difficult or impossible to act morally. Questions are ignored and moral actions suppressed. When moral integrity is compromised, nurses experience *moral distress*.

Originally described by Jameton (1984) and examined by Rodney (1988) in critical care nursing, "moral distress arises when one knows the right thing to do, but institutional restraints make it nearly impossible to pursue the right course of action" (Jameton, 1984, p.6).

The cover story of the November 1997 issue of *The Canadian Nurse* describes a situation that precipitated moral distress for nurses and became another significant event in Canadian nursing history. It explains events in a Winnipeg Hospital in 1994 when nurses' concerns regarding troubling surgical deaths were ignored. Haunted by the deaths of twelve babies, the eyes of the nurses on the cover and words of the editor, Judith Haines (1997), say it well.

When the cardiac surgery program at their institution reopens, experienced operating room nurses . . . soon recognize that something is amiss. There seem to be surgical problems, and infants begin to die . . . So the nurses try to get someone's attention. They go to their superiors, and on up the chain. Few seem to listen. At one point one of the nurses is as much as told her opinion doesn't matter, that she is a nurse, not a surgeon. Internally, though, the word is out. When a senior physician says she'll refer no more patients to the cardiac surgery program, people sit up and take notice. This is nearly 10 months later . . . Yes, if this story underlines anything, it is the damaging power relationships sometimes still at play in institutional settings, relationships that undermine nursing's voice and nurses' capacity to be true advocates for patients and families (p. 3).

In her review of this case, Laurie Hardingham (2006) notes the challenges faced by nurses to meet the expectations of their Code of Ethics and Standards of Practice. One nurse had considered warning parents but was not sure that would have helped the situation. She believed she would not be taken seriously, would have lost her job but the program would have still continued. The following excerpt from the inquest report (Sinclair 2000) places the case in the larger context of health care.

... In this context, whistle-blowing refers to the situation where a person relays information to someone outside the regular reporting process of a hospital in order to reveal something that has happened, in an attempt to bring about a more public investigation. Obviously, with the issues of confidentiality and privacy that go with medical treatment, hospital personnel cannot easily speak publicly about how a particular patient or group of patients have been treated or are being treated in a particular facility, by a particular doctor, or within a particular medical program. As well, with hospitals having put in place processes for staff members to relay their concerns about treatment, it is reasonably expected that if the proper process is used, proper steps will then be taken to address legitimate concerns . . .

Youngson had good reason to fear that her complaints would not be validated by the hospital, even if she went public with them. The problems that confronted Youngson and the other nurses in getting heard do not reflect a lack of professional responsibility on their part; rather, they appear to reflect the historically subordinate role that the nursing profession has played in our health-care system (p. 355).

When their reports regarding the unusual number of deaths went unheeded by senior officials, nurses did not feel free to take further action but instead, they questioned their own values and actions. As a result, they experienced moral distress then and may continue to carry its residue with them today. Unresolved moral distress may become *moral residue*, which Webster and Baylis (2000) describe as "that which each of us carries with us from those times in our lives when in the face of moral distress we have seriously compromised ourselves or allowed ourselves to be compromised" (p. 218).

Ann Hamric (2010) reviewed a case of moral distress experienced by a nurse in the Intensive Care Unit of an American Hospital. The nurse advocated for a patient who did not wish to be kept alive on a ventilator; but the physician insisted that the patient could still recover. A year earlier, the same nurse had requested an ethics consultation on a similar case that was eventually resolved in the physician's favour. The hospital then implemented a policy allowing only physicians or family members to request ethics consults. Physicians, who may experience moral distress when burdened with responsibility for withdrawing treatment, focus on "the survival of the few", while nurses deal with the "suffering of the many" (p.4).

Responses to moral distress and its contributing factors

Hamric (2010) describes three typical responses by nurses to moral distress recorded in the literature. The first is "a numbing of moral sensitivity and withdrawal from involvement in ethically challenging situations." The second is to leave the profession, and the third is to "resort to conscientious objection to advocate for their patients." She concludes:

An important first step in dealing with moral distress, however, is for nurses to speak up, and for other nurses, managers, administrators, and physicians to recognize and support their concerns. Those nurses most deeply concerned for their patients' welfare are precisely the ones we can't afford to lose (p. 6).

A British Columbia study (Varcoe, Pauly, Storch, Newton & Makaroff, 2012) examined nurses' perceptions of and responses to *moral distress*. Two hundred and ninety-two nurses practicing in acute care settings identified practice issues contributing to their moral distress. These included *workload, lack of leadership, witnessing unnecessary suffering, moral compromise and negative judgments by providers about patients and/or their families*. The nurses described measures taken to address these matters. Direct actions such as calling a physician to request or change an order are an integral part of the nurses' role. More creative activities included writing letters, setting up meetings to debrief situations and/or plan collective action, consulting with a professional body or ethics committee, offering to help write policy and filing incident reports. Responses to the nurses' actions included "inaction, demeaning replies, resisting and deflecting concerns, and responsive actions, a range that illustrated the contextual and relational nature of actions in the face of moral distress" (p.495).

As reported in this study, *workload* is contributing to moral distress for nurses in the current health care system. A publication by the Canadian Federation of Nurses Unions (2012) notes that in spite of numerous studies during the past 20 years, matters affecting nurses' workload and work life have not been addressed.

> Relying on the best evidence, and on the experience of frontline nurses, *Nursing Workload and Patient Care* presents a sobering look at the challenges facing our overworked nursing workforce and the ensuing effects on patients. *Nursing Workload and Patient Care* lays bare the empty promises of countless government studies while urging policy makers to fully understand the value that a nurse's education and training bring to patient care (p.1).

The report's executive summary states:

> Poor work environments continue to impact nurses' ability to provide safe care. Frequent interruptions, role confusion, limited technical and human support, lack of system integration and coordination, relentlessly increasing patient acuity, and a *lack of autonomous decision making and input into patient care decisions* continue to negatively impact nurses and the patients and families they serve. Today's nurses continue to experience high levels of burnout, absenteeism, turnover and fatigue, and lack of job satisfaction. Studies show a direct correlation between nurse satisfaction and patient satisfaction (p. 14).

Even though I am no longer in the nursing work-force, I support nurses in their ongoing struggle for satisfactory working conditions in order to provide adequate patient care. The context and nature of health care has changed but two things apparently remain constant for nurses: the *lack of autonomous decision making and input into patient care decisions* and their fortitude in working for quality health care. In June 2013, the Association of Registered Nurses of BC (2013) released a statement on Staff Mix Decision-Making and Nursing Practice that followed principles in a Canadian Nurses Association framework approved the previous year. Its fourth principle is: "Direct care nursing staff and nursing management are engaged in decision-making about the staff mix."

My most common response to situations that compromised patient care was to write letters to health care leaders, politicians and, on occasion, editors of local newspapers. Writing about matters affecting nursing practice was one way of informing and prompting action by the authorities. For example, I wrote a letter to hospital administration regarding incidents in the smoking lounge next to the psychiatric unit where I worked in the early 1990's. Since it was the only smoking lounge in the hospital, patients came, often alone or with an intravenous pole, from other units for a smoke. When a patient fell, became ill or distressed, nurses from our unit were summoned to help. We were called away from our own patients to deal with situations involving patients unknown to us. I appealed to the authorities to address the problem that was placing both patients and nurses at risk. My letter was acknowledged with a promise that the matter would be addressed.

In a different situation, when a letter to the editor about a collaborative project making the transplantation of animal organs into humans possible appeared in the *Edmonton Journal*, I wrote a letter raising questions about the ethical and social implications of xenographs (animal for human transplants) and calling for ethical review of the potential long term effects of such practices.

During my practicum in health care ethics four years earlier, I had given considerable thought to the implications of organ donation and transplantation. On one occasion, while serving as chaplain in an intensive care unit, I sat with the family of a woman being assessed for brain death and candidacy for organ donation. Members of the transplant team (sometimes referred to as "organ mongers") came to the unit to see the patient and speak with her family. The family's shock and grief regarding the loss of their loved one became clouded and confused by a suggestion that organ donation could give meaning to their loved one's death. As they struggled with their decision, the implication that death had no meaning without organ donation was troubling for me. Whatever the circumstances, grief includes remembering, honouring and finding meaning in the loss of a loved one. After pondering what their mother would have wanted, the family eventually agreed to donate her organs. When she was taken to the operating room with the venti-lator still breathing for her to ensure that her organs remained viable for transplantation, I regretted that her family was denied the opportunity to be with her as she breathed her last breath. I was also distressed by what I perceived to be subtle, yet coercive tactics to procure organs.

My intention when writing the letter to the editor in 1991 was to highlight the complexity of organ transplantation and the need to protect the integrity of both donor and recipient. Animal organ to human transplants might eliminate the concern about human donors but creates new issues. Since then, apparently because of a shortage of donors meeting brain death criteria, organs may now be taken from donors meeting cardiac death rather than brain death criteria. The practice is a source of moral distress for some health professionals. Dr. Ari Joffe (2011) questions the practice and appeals for "truthful, complete, voluntary consent to organ donation and a moratorium of the practice of organ donation after cardio circulatory death (DCD)" (p.5).[ix]

Nurses and the media: An ambivalent relationship

My letter (Schattschneider, 1991) got the attention of the Media Watch Committee of the Alberta Association of Registered Nurses. When the committee noted that my professional credentials were not published along with my name at the end of the letter, an inquiry in this regard was sent to the newspaper editor. Apparently, the paper's practice of publishing credentials of physicians (which were included with the original letter about the project) did not apply to nurses. Some years later, journalists Bernice Buresh and Suzanne Gordon (2000) were asking questions about the media's apparent indifference to nurses, and later wrote the book, *From Silence to Voice*, to encourage nurses to communicate what they know to the public. Their intention to promote nurses' visibility in the media changed when they learned that nurses are often reluctant to speak publicly about their work.

In fact, silence is part of nursing history and culture. *I see and I am silent* was the mission statement of the Nightingale School of Nursing founded in 1874 in St. Catharines, Ontario (Rankin, 1988). A directive from Florence Nightingale's address to probationers and nurses at the Nightingale School at St. Thomas Hospital emphasizes *the silent power of a consistent life.*

> A person in charge must be felt more than she is heard, not heard more than she is felt. She must fulfill her charge without noisy disputes, by *the silent power of a consistent life*, in which there is not seeming, and not hiding, but plenty of discretion. She must exercise authority without appearing to exercise it (Nightingale, 1914).

In their conversations with nurses, Buresh and Gordon found that some nurses, out of concern for the moral integrity of their profession, feared that speaking publicly could be seen as self-serving and do more harm than good.

Most health care employers have designated spokespersons for the organization, and nurses are often warned not to speak to media. I recall my own uneasiness when, with authorization by my employer, I was interviewed by newspaper reporters about health care programs that I coordinated. While these were opportunities to inform the public, there was also a chance that the reporters would misinterpret what was said and put their own spin on the stories. Even without interviewing nurses, journalists can help raise the profile of nursing by ensuring that reports about health care include references to nursing and its place in the health care system.

Nurses do raise their voices often away from the public eye (and ear), on behalf of their patients, but when their voices are silenced and nursing becomes invisible, nurses experience moral distress. Yet, many nurses find creative ways of getting the attention of the authorities. Nursing's visibility and voice are part of its moral work. The following chapter explores the relationship between health care reform in the 1990's and the invisibility of nursing.

Questions for reflection and discussion

1. What would you have done if you were one of the nurses in the Operating Room in the hospital in Winnipeg where infants were dying?

2. Give an example of moral distress in your own practice and describe how you dealt with it. What are the most helpful responses to situations causing moral distress for nurses and other health professionals?

3. Do you think the public understands nurses' work? If not, what can you and others do to change that?

4. What is your explanation for the nurses' apparent reluctance to speak publicly about their work?

Eight
Health Care Reform and the Invisible Work of Nursing

For us who nurse, our Nursing is a thing, which, unless in it
we are making progress every year, every month, every week,
take my word for it, we are going <u>back</u>.
Florence Nightingale, 1872 (Ulrich, B. (1992, p.13).

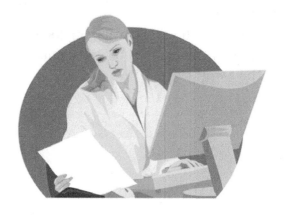

Canadian health care reform in the 1990's, driven by
economics rather than quality of patient care, was a
set-back for nursing. A network of national and provincial nursing organizations regulate nursing practice, provide professional support, represent nursing in health care planning and bargain for nurses'
working conditions. Beginning with a historical

overview of some of these organizations, this chapter describes interventions to address the impact of health care reform on nursing and allocation of health care resources. Since I was practicing in Alberta and a member of the Provincial Council for the Alberta Association of Registered Nurses when these reforms and cut-backs began, early examples are from that province. Several other examples are from British Columbia where I now live.

Professional nursing

According to the Webster dictionary, a nurse is "one specially trained to care for sick or disabled persons," but general use of the term can be confusing for the public. The College of Registered Nurses of British Columbia (2013), licensing authority for registered nurses and nurse practitioners in BC, clarifies what to expect from nurses and notes the term *nurse* is protected by law. It can only be used by a registered nurse (RN), nurse practitioner (NP), licensed practical nurse (LPN) or registered psychiatric nurse (RPN). For the most part, references to nurses in this book are referring to Registered Nurses.

The Canadian Nurses Association (CNA) represents registered nurses in national health care planning and policy development. At the same time, provincial nursing organizations regulate nursing practice to ensure that nurses are providing safe, competent and ethical nursing to the public. As a result of recent Health Professions legislation, these regulatory bodies are now referred to as *colleges*. Provincial nursing associations continue to participate in advocacy and political action on behalf of nursing.

Collective bargaining for nurses

The Canadian Nurses Association approved collective bargaining regarding salaries and working conditions for nurses in 1944. Provincial nursing associations in Quebec and British Columbia were the first to establish bargaining units. British Columbia nurses formed an independent union, British Columbia Nurses Union (BCNU), in 1981.

Alberta nurses established a bargaining unit in its professional association in 1964 and formed a separate provincial union, United Nurses of Alberta (UNA), in 1977. During the next five years, UNA members went on strike three times. In her review of the rise of nursing unions in Alberta, Janet Ross-Kerr (1998) notes:

> Conflicting ethical positions may present dilemmas for nurses where strike action is contemplated. Whether or not to stay on the job when working conditions raise questions about patient safety must be balanced with the ethical and legal duty of a nurse to care for a patient who requires nursing care (p. 280).

Working in "out of scope" positions or, as in 1982, a member of another union, the Staff Nurses Association at the University of Alberta Hospital, I did not participate in strike action. Initially, I was ambivalent about the militant union approach that conflicted with my image of nurses as caring professionals but ultimately,

I benefited from its work. The public also benefits when nursing unions advocate, not only for satisfactory working conditions for nurses, but for sufficient staff to provide safe, adequate service to the public.

Cuts in health care spending

When the Klein government in Alberta began slashing health care funding in 1993, many new nursing graduates and laid-off nurses left the country for employment elsewhere. Some have not returned. Nurses bumped into positions held by others with less seniority but often with more experience in their specialty. Individually and collectively, nurses, including the professional association and nursing unions, lobbied the government to consider the impact of these cuts on health care. As positions for registered nurses are eliminated, responsibilities increase for the remaining RNs overseeing staff, assessing patients and managing their care.

In this context, student nurses were naturally anxious about job prospects even as they dealt with the pressure of academic studies and clinical work. When a student in my mental health nursing class researched the incidence of depression and suicide amongst college students, she noted the reluctance of students to talk about the issue. Her question; *"Is all the stress, and at times, depression that student nurses experience a prerequisite for being a real nurse?"* begged the question:

"How were "real" nurses, including nursing instructors, modeling self-care, stress management and

healthy lifestyles?" Workload, student demands and competition to achieve tenure created constant pressure in the academic workplace. However, our primary responsibility was to prepare students for nursing practice and support their professional aspirations in spite of dim employment prospects.

In early 1994, I moved to a sessional nursing education position in British Columbia where health care cuts began later that year. Referred to as the era of national health care reform, the 1990's was a period of downsizing and reorganization precipitated by cuts in federal transfer payments to provinces by the Chretien government elected in October 1993. As health care reform continued, organizational structures were constantly in flux with shuffles in management and changes in lines of accountability. Much administrative time and many resources were wasted while workplace morale deteriorated.

Beginning in British Columbia, nurses across the country began job action in November 1998. An article in the national medical journal entitled, "RN= Really Neglected, angry nurses say" (Sibbald, 1999), quotes Kathleen Connors, president of the National Federation of Nurses Unions: "Nurses have been able to provide minimally necessary physical care . . . but the emotional aspects, the 'tapestry of caring' that is the essence of nursing, has suffered, and nurses are 'fed up and tired' (p.1490). Their concerns caught the attention of physicians who admitted that nurses were being "downtrodden." The quality of patient care and nurses' work life was being negatively affected by the "casualization" of the nursing workforce. New graduates and those unable to find permanent work are often forced into casual employment that does not allow for professional growth and development, enhance job satisfaction or ensure continuity of patient care. The article concludes: "RNs are in dire need of the 2Rs: respect and recognition" (p. 1491).

Ongoing challenges

Talk about cut-backs and lay-offs of nurses in the early 1990's turned into warnings about shortages the following decade. A *Nanaimo Daily News* (2000) editorial entitled: "Wake up to nursing shortages" reported that the number of nurses in Canada was declining while the average age of nurses increased. It noted that little attention is paid to nurses—the "backbone" of the health care system and warned the "backbone" is crumbling further as nurses leave the field because of stress. Nurses make up one third of the Canadian health care workforce and are an essential part of health care. Yet they are apparently considered dispensable as their job security swings back and forth with the pendulum of health care funding. It was rare but encouraging to see an editorial dedicated to the topic. Public conversations regarding health care usually focus on physician or medical care, waitlists for tests and surgical procedures; but people need to know there is much more to health care.

That same year, the book, *Critical Care: Canadian nurses speak for change*, was released. It features stories of nurses in 45 nursing specialties serving persons of all ages in a range of settings from homes, schools, specialty clinics, hospitals to war and disaster zones. Author Andre Picard (2000), *Globe and Mail* health reporter, writes:

> A theme that runs through *Critical Care* is the importance of investing not only in good, solid medical care, but also in public health (and public health nurses) to create a system that provides humane treatment for illness, and promote wellness—a concept that has been marginalized and undervalued, much as nurses have been (p. 6).

As nurses integrate the academic, scientific, technical, interpersonal and moral dimensions of their work, nursing has become highly specialized. Picard (2000) describes the apparent reservations about that specialization.

> There are two underlying fears of specialization: that nurses are somehow going to "steal" the work of doctors, and that by doing more "doctor-like" work, nurses will somehow become less caring . . .
> Caring and skills are not mutually exclusive. On the contrary, the profession of modern nursing has always consisted of caring with a scientific basis. The science, the education, has always been there, it is now just more prominent. That does not mean it has to dominate, the way it does with physicians. If anything, nurses have to strive *to elevate caring to its*

rightful place. Only then will the work of nurses be understood, and appreciated (p. 243).

To elevate caring to its rightful place, nurses, along with educators, employers and health care policy makers, need to value and affirm the nurse-patient relationship as nursing's moral foundation. Nurses who entered the profession because of its caring dimension are burning out and leaving the profession when unable to fulfill their moral commitments to their patients.

A Canadian Nurses Association (2009b) Fact Sheet explains why 250,000 nurses working on the front lines are a good investment for the health system— saving lives, promoting health and reducing costs. In spite of nurses' efforts over the past 20 years to educate the public about the vital role of nurses in health care, the status of nursing has come full circle. Nursing layoffs in the 1990's led to a shortage of nurses at the end of the decade. In spite of the education of new nurses to replace an aging nursing workforce, full-time employment for new graduates is not guaranteed. Since the downturn in the economy in 2008, new care delivery models are "reinventing the 1990's wheel" and replacing nurses with unlicensed personnel (British Columbia Nurses Union, 2013a).

Nurses continue to appeal for public support in addressing these matters. In 2012, the British Columbia Nurses Union (2012) launched a campaign, *Safe Care Now,* calling for adequate staffing levels to ensure *patient safety.*

> *Patient safety* is about applying best practices, to achieve positive health outcomes, and avoiding unsafe acts so as to reduce mortality and morbidity . . . Overburdened nurses are less able to perform the complex tasks of clinically monitoring and coordinating patient care . . .
>
> Nurses are the "backbone" of our health care system; as nursing goes, so goes the rest of the system. Their workload is multifaceted and complex. A significant factor in workload stress for hospital and community nurses is work intensity, which has increased due to shorter hospital stays and more complex health problems per patient. Work intensity escalates when hospitals are filled to capacity (p.1).

The intricacies of nurses' work are not readily apparent to the casual observer and may be discounted by health care planners and authorities.

The invisibility of nursing and the moral work of nurses

So why is nursing work seemingly invisible to so many? To shed light on the question, Pamela Bjorklund (2004) reviewed writings by nurse researchers, Joan Liaschenko from Minnesota and Patricia Rodney from British Columbia. These researchers have focused on nurses' ethical concerns, their moral work and knowledge that is often unseen except by other nurses. As a result of its "invisibility", some of that work is not factored into economic equations, which in turn has led to unseen costs. Bjorklund elaborates:

> The costs to patients were incalculable, for ultimately nurses sacrificed the invisible work of providing emotional support and systems work on patients' behalf to more visible nursing work that had been costed and thus had economic value to the institution (p.116).

In addition, even though nurses' communication and exchange of information with patients and other health care professionals is an essential part of health care, these interactions—often invisible, are undervalued. Bjorklund concludes:

> The gaze (the ethical eye of nursing) encompasses multiple forms of knowledge, some of it legitimated by the biomedical structure in which nursing is embedded, but much of it dismissed and a large part of it not even seen. The knowledge that is most important to keeping the patient central to that gaze is that which is most difficult to represent and the easiest to overlook (p.120).

Indeed, nurses' moral work includes keeping the focus on the patient.

In this digital age, our health care system relies heavily on computer data. As a result, in some situations, the nurse's role has been diminished to digital technician rather than skilled, knowledgeable, professional clinician. I wonder how novice nurses, with less time to engage with and care for patients, can develop skills and ability to make clinical judgments. When providing care, expert nurses draw on past experience, observations and knowledge of the patient. Nurses with a sense of salience practice the intuitive art of nursing by:

> selectively ignor[ing] the less important aspects of the situation (from their learned perspective) and are sensitive to nuances that might influence the more significant aspects. This view of salience ... asserts that the knower (unlike a computer) has direct access to the situation through skills, and a committed stance (Benner,1984, p. 298).

Note the distinction between the intuitive grasp of a situation and computerized interpretation of data.

After careful examination of fiscal and information based health care management inside Canadian health care reform, Marie Campbell and Janet Rankin (2006) conclude:

> We have come to recognize that nurses' consciousness is being reorganized away from their traditional standpoint in the expression of caring ... Socialized and trained to care for people, nurses are now being taught, coached and persuaded that it is their professional duty to nurse the organization (p.171).

Are health authorities paying attention to this trend? If so, who is willing to address the matter? Seemingly, political, health care management and professional power structures can easily become detached from the daily reality of those bearing the burden of health care on the front lines.

That was evident in CBC's Fifth Estate program (CBC, 2013) rating Canadian hospitals and reporting on its survey of registered nurses across the country. While 60 per cent of the respondents reported that staffing shortages were affecting patient care, 40 per cent of the nurses were experiencing burn-out. In a joint press release, The Canadian Nurses Association (2013) and the Canadian Federation of Nurses Unions expressed their determination "to ensure that the Fifth Estate's series will reignite important discussions and compel governments, providers and Canadians for work together for change."

Clearly, the nursing profession and health care system face a moral crisis. The principle *of justice* in health care ethics, when applied to the allocation of health care resources, is referred to as *distributive justice*. The egalitarian theory of justice, combining the principles of need and equality, guides nursing practice in Canada. "Just as at the level of patient care nurses should allocate their time to those they serve based on the assessment of the patients' needs, so too at the level of public policy resources government should allocate resources proportionate to needs among the population" (Yeo, Rodney, Moorhouse, & Khan (2010 b, p.302-303).

Isabelle St. Pierre (2012) argues that "nurses are in fact victims of distributive injustice when workloads exceed the capacity of the available human resources" (p.9). Are health care leaders ready to reverse this

pattern of exploitation? Nurses have a moral obligation to protect their own health and well-being while
working for the health and well-being of those whom
they serve. In turn, health care decision makers and
employers have a moral obligation to ensure that
nurses have the necessary resources to do that work.

Nursing at the crossroads

In 2009, the Canadian Nurses Association (2009 c)
released its Vision for Nursing and Health focusing
on "keeping people well by linking health to social
determinants, supporting health promotion and promoting community based care as well as acute illness
care"(p.1). The Association later set up a commission
to examine health care priorities by looking at factors,
such as housing, education, employment, access to
adequate nutrition and clean water, affecting people's
health. The National Expert Commission considered
the prevalence of chronic health conditions, growth
of Canada's aging population and health needs in
aboriginal communities. Its report (Canadian Nurses
Association, 2012a) was released in June 2012. In
order to better serve the health needs of Canadians
and ensure sustainability of the health care system,
the Commission recommends a plan of action led by
"informed, well-educated and committed nurses,"
to shift the emphasis from acute care in hospitals to
community primary care teams focusing on prevention and management of chronic illnesses.

The prospect of transforming the system to
increase its effectiveness and efficiency is appealing.

However, for nurses to be accepted as leaders of the process, entrenched attitudes and power structures need to change. Since Medicare was implemented in the 1960's, physicians, paid on a fee for service basis, have been the gatekeepers and primary entry point to the system. In 1988, medical ethicist John Thomas (1988) noted that the health care funding method reinforced the privileged status given to physicians in our society, and described the dilemma regarding payment for nurses' services. He suggested that nursing was at the crossroads and proposed an option for controlling costs:

> The effectiveness of the "high tech" approach to improved health is currently under fire. Whether people would be healthier if the cut-backs were made on esoteric medicine and redirected to improved nursing care might be a question worth exploring (p.30).

Twenty-five years later, nursing is again at the crossroads. Nurses provide care and support while assessing, informing, advocating and coordinating services for persons in a variety of settings. Although nurses' work increases the efficiency of health care, its merits are underestimated. Transformation of health care can happen only with acceptance and backing by politicians, health care authorities, physicians, nurses, other health professionals, the public and media. With nurses working within their full scope of practice, members of the public can enjoy greater access to health care that supports them in managing health problems, and physicians are better able to focus on patients' medical needs. Initial incremental changes could concentrate on patients discharged from crowded hospitals, especially elderly and other vulnerable persons with needs that surpass available family and community resources. Our ideal, and ultimately, our goal is sustainable, quality health care and optimum well-being for all.

Fifty years after walking up the front steps of the nurses' residence to launch my nursing career, I have a much deeper understanding of what it means to be a nurse. Definitions, theories, lofty aspirations and reports fall short in describing the essence of nursing. Our quest needs to move deeper to its very core, especially as we interpret it and educate new graduates for a profession that continues to evolve. Mentoring of nursing students and new graduates by experienced nurses who model the ideals of caring, patient empowerment and innovative leadership is essential for the survival and advancement of the profession.

The real meaning of nursing experienced by past and present generations will be passed on in the stories of those called to nurse (Shalof, 2008, 2009; Gordon, 2010). My own story is how my belief that nursing is at the heart of health care motivates me to ask questions and advocate for safe, ethical and compassionate care for all patients/clients. It embraces what I learned from the people who placed their trust in me as a nurse. In the end, the need to care for myself was my most important lesson—lessons to be discussed in the next chapter.

Questions for reflection and discussion

1. What is your response to these questions raised at the beginning of the chapter?

2. Is all the stress, and at times, depression that student nurses experience a prerequisite for being a real nurse?

3. How were "real" nurses and nursing instructors modeling self-care, stress management and healthy lifestyles?

4. How would you describe patient safety? What factors are essential for adequate monitoring of a patient's condition and prevention of critical incidents?

5. Name some of the "invisible aspects" of nurses' work. Do you value that work? Does it make a difference for patients/clients?

6. What does distributive justice mean to you? Give examples of situations where there is an unfair or unequal distribution of resources in our society?

7. Can you imagine a health care system led by nurses that places more emphasis on the community and value of community care? How can nurses facilitate that transition?

Nine
Nurses' Health: Balancing the Teeter-totter of Life and Work

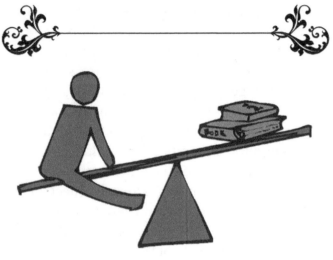

Beginning with a word from Ziggy:
Remember this . . . If you're gonna be any good to others . . .
you gotta be good to yourself once in a while!

That cartoon travelled with me for years as a reminder to maintain a balanced lifestyle. At certain crisis points in my life and career, I discovered the necessity of taking time away from the politics and tensions in the workplace to ponder my purpose and nurture my soul.

I was drawn to positions where employers welcomed

my ideas and entrusted me with projects designed to serve the needs of specific client groups. Nursing had meaning when I saw beyond daily routines to appreciate the bigger picture and importance of the work. Paradoxically, that ability was also a source of stress. Often without job security, the work's ambiguity and lack of formal structure demanded an extra amount of resilience.

Resilience is "the ability to remain strong amid ambiguity and change and is a skill that is developed and honed" (Sankey, 2005). It requires good physical and mental health. According to Edelwich & Brodsky (1980), burn-out, setting in when energy and interest wane, is:

> the progressive loss of idealism, energy, and purpose experienced by people in the helping professions as a result of the conditions of their work. Those conditions range from insufficient training to client overload, from too many hours to too little pay, from inadequate funding to ungrateful clients, from bureaucratic to political constraints to the inherent gap between aspiration and accomplishment p.14).

A review of the moral component of nurse-burnout (Cameron 1986) notes that nurses prone to burnout tend to view their work situations as threats—one such threat being moral compromise. That was the case for me when my values were seemingly under siege. One value central to my life and work as a nurse is *integrity,* a fundamental value for nursing practice.

> *Integrity* has a unique place among the values that guide nursing practice. It is more fundamental than the other values involved in nursing. Indeed, when pushed to a limit any issue involving those other values—beneficence, autonomy, truthfulness, confidentiality and justice—can also become an issue of integrity. As a concept rich in meaning, then integrity can be distinguished by four constituent features; *moral autonomy; fidelity to promise, steadfastness, and wholeness* (Yeo, et al. 2010a, p.349-350).

Moral autonomy has been discussed in earlier accounts of my quest for recognition of nurses' moral agency. Integrity is demonstrated by keeping promises "to respect patient values and choices, protect private information and confidences, and to help and not harm patients" (Yeo, et al. 2010 a, p.351). Remaining steadfast in standing up for what one believes to be right, even when circumstances work against our position, can be the ultimate test of integrity. Meanwhile, wholeness and the integrative work of self-examination, reflection, dialogue with others are essential for health and strength to face each day.

In their qualitative study of how nurses enact ethical practice, researchers use the image of nurses "navigating towards a moral horizon" (Rodney, Varcoe, Storch, McPherson, Mahoney, Brown, Pauly, Hartrick & Starzomksi (2002). The "horizon" metaphor represents the "good" towards which nurses are navigating. Although currents of resistance within the moral climate of the workplace might affect that journey, nurses reported that ethics education, professional and collegial support helped keep them on course.

For me, going to work sometimes felt like heading into a storm to be tossed about by the waves and beaten against the rocks. I looked forward to returning to the safety of home where a poster on the inside of my apartment door read: *Ships in a harbor are safe but that is not what ships are for.* On better days in calmer waters, my spirits were lifted by comradeship with colleagues collaborating to improve the health and quality of life of the persons seeking our support and care.

Burn-out is characterized by detachment and over-involvement, but over-involvement is also a sign of co-dependence. It is a pattern of interpersonal interaction rooted in low self-esteem and often associated with addictive organizations or families (Beattie, 1987). Co-dependents care for and control others rather than care for themselves. Co-dependence is learned in situations where people are encouraged to deny feelings or problems, keep secrets, be perfect and discouraged from thinking for themselves. Health professionals may unconsciously adopt habits reinforced by the demands and rigid rules in health care bureaucracies. Controlling managers try to please everyone and avoid open discussion of issues. (Cauthorne-lindstrom & Hrabe, 1990; Arnold, 1990).

The Serenity Prayer, commonly used in 12 step addiction recovery programs, acknowledges the need to find the balance between control and change.

God, grant me the serenity to accept the things I cannot change, courage to change the things I can, and wisdom to know the difference.

Without fully understanding its significance, I posted the Serenity Prayer in my office during my first management job and kept it somewhere in view over the following years. It became a watchword as I longed for serenity and wisdom, especially when needing to accept that some challenges were beyond my control.

I earned a reputation for being a reliable and conscientious nurse but some suggested I was overly zealous, sensitive and cared too much. A colleague in management even warned me that I would not advance in the organization if I kept using the word *share*. Admittedly, I took my work seriously, valued team work and did not want to be nursing if the flame of my passion and enthusiasm was extinguished.

In a graduate seminar attempting to illustrate an ethic of care in diagram format, the theoretical discussion struck me as disconnected from the day-to-day experiences of nurses. The previous evening at work, I dealt with an out-of-control psychotic patient requiring sedation. Shaken by the incident, I inadvertently pricked myself with the needle used for the injection. (Nurses are warned to take precautions to prevent such incidents and the possibility of being infected with HIV or hepatitis.) The patient was still on my mind the following morning when I blurted, "We can't draw it—we just do it!"

For me, caring was a moral responsibility and part

of my vocation. It was one of my greatest strengths but was also my greatest weakness when concern for patients and zeal to do the right thing affected my health and communication with others. I often blamed myself when workplace relationships became strained but eventually learned that, while I needed to take responsibility for my own conduct, the work-place culture also sets the tone for interpersonal interactions. Ethical practice is facilitated in support-ive workplace environments that foster open commu-nication without fear of repercussions.

Mental health: a priority

Becoming less resilient to change and stress in mid-life, I took time off when working in a city far from my prairie roots. It was unusual for me to take sick leave, but the hospital staff health nurse reassured me that my reaction to the particular stresses on the job was normal but significant enough to warrant attention. Even in the city, one of my survival mechanisms was to walk or bike in a nearby park—exercise and green space helped reground me.

Eventually some years later, the cumulative stress progressed from burn-out to clinical depression. Lack of sunlight during short winter days and work in win-dowless offices was likely a contributing factor given that sunshine affects the level of serotonin, a mood altering hormone in the brain. Seasonal Affective Disorder (SAD), or "winter blues" in its milder form, is characterized by "feeling blue", low energy, irri-tability and difficulty concentrating. It is common amongst shift workers who see little if any daylight during their working hours (Canadian Mental Health Association, 2013).

Stress and depression amongst health care workers is more common than many want to admit. After all, aren't we expected to manage stress? I believed that I could manage my own stress until medical treatment relieved my symptoms of chronic fatigue, irritability, depressed mood and hopelessness. One of my nurse colleagues even expressed surprise that I would admit to being depressed, given that such an admission could affect my career. Even in the health care workplace, people with mental health problems may be stigmatized. However, perpetuating the secrecy, denial and shame about these matters is not helpful for anyone.

Reflecting on the suicide of a nursing colleague early in her career, Louise Bradley (2010), RN and CEO of the Mental Health Commission of Canada, urges nurses to open up about mental illness so that people can get the help they need. *The Canadian Nurse* (2010, October) journal feature article about fatigue includes stories by nurses on the front lines. A section titled *Fatigue in the news* includes the distressing headline from the *Montreal Gazette* on August 14, 2010: *Nurses' union sounds alarm over suicides: Quebec City records four in 18-month span*. Surely, it is time to address the troubling reality of nurse suicide.

In the professional journal for British Columbia nurses, Bergen and Fisher (2003) report: "The combination and interaction of systemic and traumatic stresses place registered nurses at a high risk of suffering from serious negative stress effects in the areas of physical, emotional, cognitive, behavioral and interpersonal well-being" (p. 13). It points out nurses' responsibility to maintain physical, mental and emotional health, but that can be difficult in stressful work situations. The Fitness to Practice document of the Registered Nurses Association of B.C. also highlighted the need for managers to be "more aware of risk factors, mechanisms and effects of workplace systemic and traumatic stress" (p. 15).

According to the Canadian Broadcasting Corporation (2006), in the National Survey of Work and Health of Nurses, 31 percent of the nurses reported "a high level of psychological strain"—more than most Canadian workers. More than 50 percent of the nurses took time off the previous year for physical illness and 10 percent were off work for mental health reasons. About 9 percent of nurses, both male and female, had experienced depression in the previous year compared to 7 percent of women and 4 percent of men in the general population.

The nursing profession is especially concerned about the impact of *nurse fatigue* on nursing and patient safety. The Canadian Nurses Association (2010) Position Statement: *Taking Action on Nurse Fatigue* defines nurse fatigue as:

> A subjective feeling of tiredness that is physically and mentally penetrative. It ranges from tiredness to exhaustion, creating an unrelenting overall condition that interferes with individuals' physical and cognitive

ability to function to their normal capacity . . . CNA declares that factors in today's health system environment contribute to nurse fatigue, including increased worker stress, increased workload, understaffing, increased expectations from patients and families, high levels of patient acuity, unexpected emergencies with staffing or patients, sensory overload, functionally disorganized workplaces (p.1).

The document acknowledges that nurses experience moral distress when the workplace culture does not support open acknowledgement of nurse fatigue as a patient and staff safety issue. Nevertheless, it reminds nurses of their commitment to safe, compassionate, competent, ethical care and ethical obligation to maintain fitness to practice. The statement identifies systemic, organizational and individual responsibilities to prevent and manage nurse fatigue.

A later Canadian Nurses Association (2012b) Fact Sheet on Nurse Fatigue identifies the negative impact of fatigue on nurses' physical and mental health, lifestyle and relationships. It notes that "fatigue is a factor for 26 per cent of nurses who are considering leaving the profession" (p.1).

In her dissertation, *Fatigue and Nurses' Perspective of Working the Night Shift*, Carol Rocker (2012) notes the ethical dilemma faced by health care leaders "balancing safe patient care and health care costs with that of healthy nighttime workforce" (p.110). While nurses have to take responsibility for managing their own level of fatigue, Rocker concludes that "Leaders also need to share the responsibility of reducing fatigue in the workforce, together increasing patient safety and adequate staffing levels" (p.125). Rocker's findings confirm a relationship between fatigue and nurses either looking for work without night shifts or leaving the profession.

While nurse fatigue is a consequence of excessive demands and insufficient rest, a variety of terms describe health care workers' stress. Not to be confused with the physical and mental exhaustion of nurse fatigue, *compassion fatigue* describes the phenomenon of being tired of caring. An Alberta study (Austin, Goble, Leir, & Byrne, 2009) reports that the term came into use in the 1990's to describe the social concept of public indifference to appeals for aid for disaster victims. Compassion fatigue now also applies to personal, psychological disengagement of helping professionals in their care-giving relationships. Quantitative forms of measuring practice have created a culture that discourages empathy, diminishes ethical practice and places workers at risk for compassion fatigue. The review of the nurses' experiences of compassion fatigue concludes that:

> Compassion fatigue does not result from over-engagement with patients or the over-expression of the professional's compassion, but rather compassion fatigue seems to emerge when professional-patient engagement is not supported, nor valued as an integral part of nursing practice (p. 210).

Sabo (2011) views it on a continuum of occupational stress that also includes burnout and vicarious traumatization. Jan Spilman (2013), Compassion Fatigue Specialist in British Columbia, links trauma with compassion fatigue, which she defines as:

> the natural negative consequence of working with people or animals or a wounded planet that are suffering or traumatized. Symptoms of posttraumatic stress (PTS) culminating in a diminished capacity for, or interest in, being empathic with others' suffering and disengagement from care recipients.

Spilman believes that the recognition and healing of primary and secondary traumatic stress is essential to recover from compassion fatigue. Wounds such as cynicism, a disrupted world view, heightened anxiety, alienation and guilt are invitations to spiritual awakening through story-telling, mindfulness meditation or centering prayer, expressive arts, movement practices such as yoga and dance, gathering with faith community, and connection with nature.

Although the surge of interest in these matters is encouraging, more research and administrative initiatives are necessary to address factors affecting the health and moral integrity of nurses. Furthermore, critical incidents involving violence, trauma, injury and sudden death compound stress already experienced by health care professionals. Workers are then at risk for subsequent health problems including post-traumatic stress disorder (PTSD), a condition added to the American psychiatric association's *Diagnostic and Statistical Manual of Mental Disorders* in 1980. It describes the response to a traumatic event outside the range of usual human experience such as war, violence, accidents and natural disasters.

When three children died in a house fire in a northern community, I was invited to meet with hospital staff for a debriefing, but at that time, was unfamiliar with the guidelines developed for that purpose. I wanted to know more so, on my return south, attended a Critical Incident Debriefing workshop organized by emergency workers who treated the casualties of the 1987 Edmonton tornado. It opened up new appreciation for the impact of trauma on health care workers but also expanded my understanding of the connections between anyone's experiences of trauma and their health status. When critical incidents are acknowledged and dealt with, people are less likely to develop post-traumatic stress disorder.

Ultimately, in keeping with Ziggy's remarks quoted at the beginning of this chapter, if we're going to be able to care for others, we need to care for ourselves. I do not pretend to be a role model for self-care but am open to sharing what I have learned. Nursing is a vocation that requires commitment, sensitivity, endurance and a suitable disposition. Nurses are free to choose an area of practice compatible with their interests and aptitudes. When able to achieve their professional goals, they are more likely to be enthusiastic about their work.

However, excessive workload and lack of support

from management and peers can easily stifle enthusiasm and trap workers in untenable situations. Even
though registered nurses share common knowledge,
skills and standards, their specialized knowledge and
clinical skills often apply to a specific area of practice.
Therefore, the movement of nurses from one area to
another without adequate orientation and mentoring
also contributes to their stress and burnout.

For those who "head into the storm" every day to
make a difference as a nurse, I offer these thoughts
about self-care.

1) Have Realistic Expectations

While you ought to be free to dream and imagine
an ideal world, it helps to moderate your expectations to match the reality and constraints in
health care workplaces without compromising
your moral integrity. Do not expect to be thanked
or congratulated for doing a good job. For the most
part, health care professionals do their work without fanfare. While it helps when clients or employers acknowledge your work, one needs to validate
one's own efforts.

2) Set Personal Limits and Professional Boundaries

Set limits for yourself and, in turn, respect others'
boundaries. Job descriptions, along with supervisor
and peer feedback, help define the limits of nurses'
work. However, nurses also need to set their own
personal limits, know when they've done their best,
given enough and not be driven by guilt or need for

approval. Choose causes that (depending on your position) are priorities in ensuring your own health and safety in the workplace, achieving quality service for clients and optimum health in the community, effective management of staff or best learning opportunities for students. Trying to respond to all the issues can be overwhelming and self-defeating. Find a way to relate and care for your patient without becoming part of that person's life forever. Practice "being present" to the patient and letting go as you move on. A certain level of detachment is necessary in order to do this work.

3) Maintain a Balanced Lifestyle

Ensure adequate rest, fresh air, exercise, recreation, healthy nutrition for yourself. Nurture your relationships with family. Do not allow your work to intrude into these relationships or expect your family to understand your work issues. Instead, cultivate friendships with colleagues and folk with common values who can relate to your workplace experiences and stresses. Stimulate your mind and expand your interests to include matters outside of health care. Do not take yourself too seriously. Allow yourself to laugh. Grieve your losses and disappointments and find healthy ways to express your anger. Avoid using drugs or alcohol to manage stress.

4) Nurture supportive relationships at work

Peer support in the workplace is so important especially when crises arise. Value and validate one another. If you become isolated from your peers, talk with someone you can trust about your experience. That person can also validate and support you and boost your self-esteem. In turn, stand up for colleagues who are treated badly. Continue learning and keep connected with professional networks. It is good to be informed about resources and developments within the profession.

5) **Take time out to:**
Reflect on the questions and meaning of your life and work. Celebrate and honour the sacred trust that your patients place in you. Acknowledge and seek help from your higher power—nurture your soul. Connect with nature and enjoy its wonder. Play and delight in the laughter of children. Seek professional help when wearing down under the load.

Balancing the physical, intellectual and emotional demands of nursing work is an ongoing challenge and responsibility for nurses. Yet, without support and a self-care regimen, nurses can become exhausted, cynical and disengage from their patients. When the burden of care is compounded by moral distress, some nurses will leave the profession. Nurses need to care for themselves because they are, first of all, human beings.

The time has come for the nursing profession to acknowledge and openly address nurses' health as a professional issue. While nurse unions advocate for safe and healthy workplaces (British Columbia Nurses

Union, 2013b), the profession as a whole can foster a worldview of nursing that promotes health for nurses for the sake of their own wholeness, not only for the sake of their patients. When networking with the medical profession regarding disruptive behaviour by physicians, I was privileged to meet physician champions of the physician health movement. The medical profession (Canadian Medical Association, 2003) offers physician health services to physicians dealing with health matters affecting their fitness to practice.

The British Columbia Nurses Union (2013c) Licensing, Education and Practice Program recently implemented the Early Intervention Health Program to assist nurses with mental health and addiction problems. According to the highlights of the June 2012 meeting of provincial coordinators of the Ontario Nurses Association (2012), that union is collaborating with other Ontario nursing organizations in planning a health program for nurses who have addictions and mental health problems. Such initiatives will bring these matters out of the shadows and lead the way for nursing organizations across the country. Nurse Health programs could include matters pertaining to psychological health and safety in the health care workplace, which is discussed in the next chapter.

Questions for reflection and discussion
1. What is the most stressful and/or satisfying part of your work?
2. How do you balance the "teeter-totter of life and work"?

3. How do 12-hour shifts affect nurses' health, quality of life and ability to provide safe patient care?
4. What strategies for self-care work best for you?
5. Do you agree that health care professionals have a moral responsibility to ensure their fitness to practice? What is the responsibility of the profession and the employer in this regard?

Ten
Psychological Health and Safety in the Health Care Workplace

As hazards and risk factors are identified in workplaces, standards and regulations for occupational health and safety evolve. In health care, these programs have often focused on prevention of back injuries or exposure to toxic substances. Employee *psychological health and safety* has become a major concern in the twenty-first century and is being addressed by the Mental Health Commission of Canada (2012).

Psychological health and safety in the workplace includes the respectful treatment of employees with mental illness and attention to factors threatening workers' security and emotional well-being. Health care workers may be the targets of abuse—both overt and covert violence perpetrated by the public, patients, families, and yes, even colleagues. Nurses are at risk—not only from encounters with confused or distraught patients or exposure to infectious disease, but from toxic work environments. Workplace conduct and interpersonal relationships affect the quality of patient care, workplace morale and employee health and safety. Overall, it is a moral matter.

A study of nurses' experience of violence in Alberta and British Columbia Hospitals found that 46% of the nurses surveyed had experienced abuse in the previous five shifts (Duncan, Hyndman, Estabrooks, Hesketh, Humphrey & Wong, 2001). Five types of abuse were identified: physical assault, threat of assault, emotional abuse, verbal sexual harassment and sexual assault. Noting the high percentage (70%) of nurses who did not report the abuse, the authors question if it reflects an acceptance of the culture of violence in hospitals. I wonder how many nurses did not report the violence because they feared possible backlash or thought their complaint would not be taken seriously.

Over 35% of the incidents involved emotional abuse such as hurtful attitudes or remarks, insults, gestures or humiliation before the work team. While over one third of the emotional abuse was attributed to patients and families, approximately another third of the reported incidents were perpetrated by coworkers, including physicians. Discussing their findings in a health policy journal, the authors recommend that emotional abuse be included in hospital violence prevention policies (Hesketh, Duncan, Estabrooks, Reimer, Giovannetti, Hyndman, & Acorn, 2003).

Emotional abuse is a form of *bullying*, but these researchers avoid using the term that rarely appears in Canadian nursing literature. *Horizontal violence* is an accepted description of this type of behaviour in nursing but since it can be justified and normalized as oppressed group behaviour, authors of an Australian paper (Hutchinson, Jackson, Vickers, & Wilkes. (2006) reject the term. Instead, they urge the nursing profession to practice critical thinking and action by examining bullying from the perspective of power within the organization.

A British study of nursing students' experiences of bullying concludes:

> Bullying, and its effects on self-esteem, is perpetuated by practices within nursing. This situation will only be changed if nurses and educators transform their practice and the context in which bullying occurs. Otherwise, each new generation of nurses will continue to be socialized into negative practices which undermine both their own feelings of self-worth and standards of nursing care (Randle, 2003, p.395).

The report's author later collaborated in an informative article (Randle, Stevenson, & Grayling. (2007) about strategies for changing a workplace culture that quietly supports bullying.

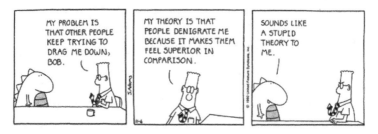

Bullying tactics include undermining or sabotaging someone's work, spreading rumours, belittling the target's ideas, abilities and contributions, verbally or physically attacking the target. When the conduct of the bully who may feel inadequate or insecure is not addressed, the target (often a conscientious, competent employee) is worn down and may be forced to leave the workplace.

Whatever we call it, bullying is more than a single event; it is a pattern of behaviours that intimidate or humiliate the target. Barbara Coloroso (2002) has written about bystanders who stand by, apparently aware but choosing not to get involved, when witnessing bullying in the school yard or workplace. When bystanders set aside their own fears of backlash or need for approval by the perpetrator, they are in the best position to break the cycle. In the absence of information from bystanders, reports by bullies and perpetrators can become a futile exercise of one person's word against that of the other. Disruptive behaviour, such as bullying, is most easily recognized by its effect on workplace morale.

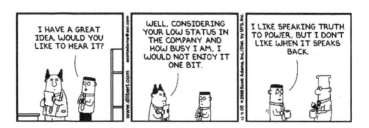

These behaviours are common amongst women who tend to use relational aggression to hurt others. According to Cheryl Dellasega (2009), a nurse and professor of Humanities and Women's Studies, *"relational aggression, a type of bullying, refers to the use*

of psychological and social behaviours rather than physical violence to cause harm" (p. 52-53). Dellasega (2005, 2011) writes about this phenomenon among women in *Mean Girls Grown Up:* and among hospital nurses in *When Nurses Hurt Nurses: Recognizing and Overcoming the Cycle of Bullying.*

Mooney (2005) reflects on how the feminist movement emphasized differences between men and women, but failed to acknowledge differences between women or prepare them for changing roles in competitive workplaces. How do women collaborate and compete at the same time? Noting that lessons about healthy relationships can be learned from athletic competition, Mooney (2005) states:

> In the workplace, rules can be hazier, competition less openly sanctioned, winners and losers less clearly cut. But in talking with so many women, I did find basic principles of athletic competition—communication, fortitude, teamwork, trust—consistently echoed in the stories of those who had successfully worked out their differences on the job (p.113).

Mobbing, a form of psychological harassment, was identified in 1980 by Swedish psychologist Heinz Leymann, who treated mobbing targets experiencing Post Traumatic Stress Disorder. Kenneth Westhues (2002), a University of Waterloo professor with an interest in mobbing in the academic environment, writes:

> ... the worst kind of harm most Canadians have to
> fear at work is the kind that arises from faulty human
> relations, some kind of glitch in how people treat one
> another. Montreal researcher Hans Selye won the
> Nobel Prize for Medicine in 1964, for the best sin-
> gle-word description of today's main workplace ills;
> stress ... Mobbing can be understood as the stressor
> to beat all stressors. It is an impassioned, collective
> campaign by co-workers to exclude, punish, and
> humiliate a targeted worker. Initiated most often by
> a person in a position of power or influence, mobbing
> is a desperate urge to crush and eliminate the target
> (p.3-4).

A coroner's inquest into the 1999 Ottawa Transpo
shooting rampage, when five people died, brought
the problem of workplace bullying into the open in
Canada. In this case, the shooter had been mobbed
by co-workers who ridiculed him for his stutter. The
inquest recommended legislation to prevent workplace violence and workplace policies to address
violence and harassment (Canada Safety Council,
2004).

Since then, four provinces (Quebec, Ontario,
Saskatchewan and British Columbia) have passed
legislation to address this covert form of violence
also referred to as psychological or personal harassment (Bullyfree BC, 2012). Most recently, changes in
the British Columbia Workers Compensation Act on
July 1, 2012 enables WorkSafeBC to deal with claims
involving mental disorders (eg. anxiety, depression)

caused by workplace stressors including workplace bullying and harassment. Occupational Health and Safety policies, developed by WorkSafeBC (2013) to help workers, employers and supervisors prevent and address workplace bullying and harassment, went into effect on November 1, 2013.

My research to learn more about this phenomenon began in 2000, a year after the murder of my brother, a physician in northern Alberta. Another physician, who ultimately was convicted of manslaughter, had lost his hospital privileges five years earlier when he declined to sign a code of conduct. He had disrupted the workplace by refusing to see patients when called, intimidating staff and threatening to have them fired or to sue the hospital board or other physicians when confronted about his behaviour. In my preparation of a paper about disruptive behaviour for a physician health conference in 2002, I found the following description helpful:

> Disruptive physicians pose special problems. They create situations in which patients are dissatisfied, staff and colleagues reach their wits' end, and administrators feel paralyzed, ... Often such doctors deny to themselves or to others the wrongful nature of their actions. They need to externalize responsibility ... by blaming coworkers, administrators, working conditions, patients, or other events. They resist effective confrontation by setting up covert threats of retaliation or even self-harm. They may overtly use their powerful positions or personalities to silence

perceived criticism. They resist the monitoring of their behaviour by challenging the authority of those who order it and by finding loopholes in the behavioral requirement. Commonly, they are so sensitive to criticism that any intervention attempt tends to heighten shameful feelings, to which they respond with more problematic behaviour. (Glendel, 2000, p.143)

I began advocating for reform in the medical profession's management of disruptive behaviour and published an article (Magnussen, 2003) and book (Magnussen, 2006) telling my brother's story. Disruptive behaviour by physicians has affected nursing practice for years and is finally getting attention within the medical profession (Rosenstein, 2002; Puddester, 2008; College of Physicians and Surgeons of Alberta, 2010).

I also talked with colleagues about our experiences of this type of behaviour in health care workplaces. It was good to have a name (or names) for a phenomenon we had personally witnessed, sometimes as targets, but had not understood. I recalled times when my work had been undermined and one occasion when a colleague warned me to "watch my back." I wondered when nursing leaders would acknowledge and address a matter affecting the health and retention of nurses.

Mary Ferguson-Pare (2008), president of the Registered Nurses Association of Ontario, writes about a gathering when nurses told stories of bullying and verbal abuse of students and other nurses. "In some instances, students were so frustrated by some of their clinical placement experiences that they are giving up before they even graduate. Others are throwing in the towel within three years of beginning their practice." She draws attention to an updated version of a position paper addressing these matters and appeals to members to refrain from this behaviour. "Remember, we need each other. We must choose to share the gift of respect with each other" (p.5).

In a report prepared for WorkSafeBC, nurse researcher Henderson (2010) describes hospital and community nurses' perceptions of how violence affected their ability to do their job and feel "safe, healthy and supported in the workplace". Violence was defined as "verbal harassment, sexual assault and physical assault as well as more subtle forms of abuse such as threatening, bullying and demeaning behaviour towards the nurse". Nurses reported experiencing or observing verbal abuse directed at themselves or a colleague from patients, relatives and/or visitors on a daily basis. They acknowledged their lack of preparation for anticipating aggression and de-escalating agitated people, lack of knowledge of policies or protocols regarding workplace violence and felt that reporting violent incidents was 'generally a waste of time'.

Nurses in the study recognized that actions by health care personnel may contribute to the escalation of violent incidents. One nurse suggested that they should spend more time talking with families and added: "I look at the time we spend in front of that computer and the managers, it's management by computer now, you know, at times I think that time would be better spent {with the patient}."

Henderson (2010) explains why health care policy makers are replacing 'zero-tolerance policies' with best practices in anticipating and de-escalating violent incidents:

> Zero tolerance policies tended to reinforce staff becoming more militant and eventually defining any negative communication as violent. Instead, researchers are coming to a consensus that better use of empathetic communication, active listening and improved assessment techniques regarding people's emotional responses to the situations in which they find themselves, might help defuse a lot of incidents before they occur.

In response to these identified concerns, Henderson developed a staff education DVD on workplace violence. She also notes that other researchers identified the prevalence of violence between workers:

> At the same time as the overall level of violence against workers in health settings is being acknowledged, there continues to be an increase in troubling reports of horizontal violence and bullying between professional groups and between co-workers.

Some writers, including Carol Rocker (2008), stress the need to address bullying in order to retain nurses. Nurse researchers Laschinger, Leiter, Day and Gilen (2009) interviewed 612 nurses from health care settings in eastern Canada and found links between workplace incivility and burnout on factors affecting retention of nurses; that is, job satisfaction, organizational commitment and turnover intentions.

A British Columbia study (Houshmand, O'Reilly, Robinson & Wolff, 2012) applied a deontic model (relating to moral obligation) to consider how employees perceived treatment in the workplace. Studying the impact of bullying on nursing staff turnover in 41 hospital units, it found that workers who were not targeted by bullies were just as likely to want to leave the workplace. It concludes that "Simply working in an aggressive environment can lead to turnover intentions because bullying represents a severe moral transgression that creates an abstract sense of moral uneasiness" (p.9). That uneasiness reflects the value nurses place on respectful and moral conduct in the workplace. When trust is violated, worker's integrity, health and safety are at risk.

Cynthia Clark (2010), an American nursing professor, emphasizes that nurses have an important role in ensuring civility and respect in nursing work and educational settings. She notes American boards of nursing are monitoring nursing programs for incivility; and the Joint Commission (which accredits and certifies health care organizations in the United States) has set a new leadership standard for appropriate conduct in accredited health care organizations. Defining *incivility* as "rude or disruptive behaviour that may result in psychological or physiological distress for the people involved, and if left unaddressed, may progress into threatening situations," Clark (2010) warns: "We must address these lesser acts of incivility before they reach a tipping point and degenerate into much worse situations that are irreversible" (p. 4).

Strategies for Restoring and preserving trust in the health care workplace

According to the Great Place to Work Institute (2012), **trust** that is demonstrated by organizational respect, fairness and credibility creates a great place to work.

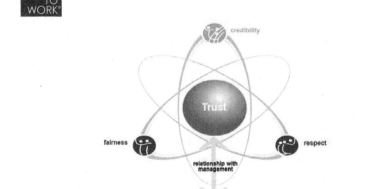

Used with permission from Great Place to Work ® Institute

Workplace bullying violates trust in relationships and jeopardizes the well-being of the organization, its employees and clients. The best way to restore trust in the workplace is to create a work environment and culture where leaders demonstrate trustworthiness and respect, and expect similar conduct by employees. All stakeholders recognize disruptive/bullying behaviour and perpetrators are held accountable.

Bullying flourishes when it is ignored or discounted. Bystanders may be conned or fear being targeted by the bully. Managers may not believe the target or want to get involved; may be intimidated by the bully; or be colluding with or even **be** the bully. Employee assistance counselors are apparently powerless to intervene since they are employed by the organization that may be enabling the bullying.

Even as targets' self-confidence and health deteriorate, they may be victimized further when blamed for the problem. Bullying targets need to confide in someone they trust in order to review and identify patterns in their experiences. Hopefully, astute bystanders can corroborate their observations, reassure targets that it is not their fault and join them in documenting critical incidents. When episodes of bullying are documented and indicate a pattern, the situation warrants attention and intervention.

Our ultimate goal is prevention—prevention of unnecessary stress, trauma and drastic outcomes by promoting safe, healthy workplaces, intervening early and addressing various forms of harassment, bullying and violence. Responding to a Statistics

Canada study reporting that in 2004, one in five violent incidents (including physical assault, sexual assault and robbery) occurred in the victim's workplace, Jessie Callaghan from the Canadian Centre for Occupational Health and Safety (Canadian Press, Ottawa (2007). recommends a preventive approach in address behaviours such as verbal abuse or psychological harassment before the situation escalates. (The Canadian Centre for Occupational Health and Safety (2009) has published a guide for developing a workplace violence prevention program).

Research practitioners at the Centre for Applied Research in Mental Health and Addiction (CARMHA, 2012) at Simon Fraser University developed and produced (with funding from Great West Life Centre for Mental Health in the Workplace) an online tool for the evaluation of psychosocial risks in the workplace. The *Guarding Minds at Work* program includes a survey that can be given to an entire workforce. The Centre also collaborated with the Mental Health Commission of Canada (2012) in developing an Action Guide to help employers protect the psychological (mental) health and safety of employees. Since then, a voluntary national standard for Psychological Health and Safety in the workplace (Mental Health Commission of Canada, 2013) has been proposed. These initiatives may identify and address practices that support workplace bullying.

Education programs that include discussion of acceptable and unacceptable workplace conduct help health care professionals recognize behaviour patterns that violate trust in the workplace. Only then can professional codes of conduct and ethics, policies and position statements be internalized and change behaviour. Significantly, the Canadian Nurses Association (2008) Code of Ethics includes reference to respect and trust. In the section on *Preserving Dignity*, the Code states:

> Nurses treat each other, colleagues, students and other health-care workers in a respectful manner, recognizing the power differentials among those in formal leadership positions, staff and students. They work with others to resolve differences in a constructive way.

In the section on *Promoting Justice*, it states:

> Nurses refrain from judging, labeling, demeaning, stigmatizing and humiliating behaviours toward persons receiving care, other health-care professionals and each other.
>
> Nurses do not engage in any form of lying, punishment or torture or any form of unusual treatment or action that is inhumane or degrading. They refuse to be complicit with such behaviours. They intervene, and then report such behaviours.
>
> Nurses support a climate of trust that sponsors openness, encourages questioning the status quo and supports those who speak out to address concerns in good faith.

+TRUTH ME(R)CY VE(G)AN+
·555· =

Hazel J. Magnussen

Workplace conduct that demonstrates and supports respectful and trusting relationships is central to the entire health care enterprise. Therefore, when violent or bullying behaviour occurs, it ought to be of concern to all stakeholders. Politicians, administrators, human resource personnel, professional associations, employee unions and the community at large need to collaborate in addressing this blight on health care. Employers have good reason to address this problem, given the economic price they pay in sick time, disability claims, grievances and even lawsuits. However, the greater cost is the loss of excellent, yet demoralized workers who give their best but without organizational support, have no choice but to move on.

Systemic change to restore and preserve trust in the health care workplace requires collaboration by the following persons and organizations:

- Workers encouraging and supporting each other in their day to day work and times of crisis.
- Managers and administrators providing leadership in developing and implementing policies and protocols for reporting and monitoring violent and disruptive behaviour in the workplace.
- Professional regulatory organizations setting standards, monitoring and holding persons accountable for unprofessional conduct.
- Labour unions monitoring and advocating for safe and healthy workplaces.

- Educational institutions modeling and instilling values of respect, discipline, care and encouraging critical thinking and ethical relationships in classroom and clinical settings.
- Politicians, governments and health boards ensuring that employment standards and workplace policies address these matters seldom visible to the public eye.
- Communities valuing and encouraging health care workers serving the public often at great cost to themselves.

The restoration of trust in the health care workplace will help form moral communities that ensure the psychological health and safety of its workers.

Questions for reflection/discussion

1. Have you observed or experienced the forms of violence and/or bullying identified in this chapter? If so, what was your response?
2. How well informed are employees and leaders in the health care workplace about workplace bullying (or whatever you want to call it)?
3. What can you do to promote psychological health and safety in your workplace? In other organizations to which you belong?

Eleven
Walking the Labyrinth: Journey to the Centre

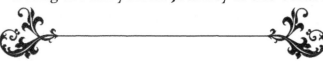

I will lead the noble soul into the wilderness—
there I will speak into her heart.
Meister Eckhart (quote from Hosea 2:14)

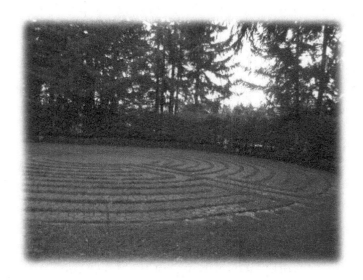

A discussion of the moral work of nursing would not be complete without reflections on its spiritual dimension. For many nurses, moral and spiritual work and care are inextricably linked. Nevertheless, spirituality may be invisible to persons unfamiliar or uncomfortable with matters pertaining to the soul. In this chapter, I reflect on the meaning of spirituality and how it and events in my life and career were intertwined.

Rolheiser (1999), an Oblate priest and spiritual writer, writes that:

> There is within us a fundamental dis-ease, an unquenchable fire that renders us incapable, in this life, of ever coming to full peace. This desire lies at the center of our lives, in the marrow of our bones, and in the deep recesses of the soul ... Spirituality is ultimately, about what we do with that desire. (p.3,5)

My desire to serve others led me to become a nurse and set the direction for my life. Before long, I knew with certainty that nursing is spiritual work. Spiritual care is treating others with respect and honouring their stories, relationships and religious practices. It embraces the mystery of life and existence of a higher power, tends to one's own and the patient's inner spirit, and reaches out to others along the way.

Spirituality is the essence of who we are and it is deepened in "wilderness experiences" of suffering. Spiritual care is therefore an integral part of health care. Nurses are often in the best position to respond to people's unspoken longings and fears but, if out of touch with their own spiritual needs, may be blind to those of others. Nurses talk about *care* but rarely speak about *compassion*—a word, derived from Latin, *paticum*, which means *to suffer with*. Sister Simone Roach (1992) draws on Henri Nouwen's writings in her description of this spiritual and, for some, radical form of caring:

Compassion is a relationship, lived in solidarity with the human condition, sharing the joys, sorrows, pain and accomplishments. Compassion involves a simple, unpretentious presence to each other, a gift that we seem to have lost even as we have developed sophisticated techniques in our efforts to acquire it ... For as Noewen insists, we do not acquire compassion by advanced skills and techniques. According to his analysis, we receive compassion as a totally gratuitous gift (p.59).

After reading an article reviewing the nursing literature regarding the question: "Why is it so hard to talk about spirituality?" (Molzahn & Shields, 2008), I was heartened by an apparent renewed interest in the subject. The belief that it is the clergy's responsibility and a lack of language and education about spirituality inhibit nurses from talking about it. They are afraid of offending others and hesitant to raise spiritual matters in a science based health care model. Spiritual care may seem irrelevant when fiscal and time constraints prevail.

Discussing the dilemmas and possibilities of spirituality and spiritual care, three nursing professors (Bruce, McDonald & McIntyre, 2006) state:

> If we accept the assumption that no single expression of spirituality can embrace all human experience, then it cannot be anticipated that nurse will know how to recognize or interpret the multiple possible expressions of spirituality or spiritual

need. However, what nurses can do (and often do very well) is enter into and engage with the unique experiences of patients . . . Nurses can be willing and able to engage patients with spiritual awareness about values, beliefs, and their experiences of illness (p.441-442).

When I took time off for pastoral care training in the middle of my career, my first lesson was learning that pastoral care or spiritual care is about *being* rather than *doing*. As a nurse, I was used to doing something for my patient's pain or other troublesome symptoms so I needed to learn to just **be** with the patient. I applied much of that learning to my nursing practice in the following years, but sometimes longed for the freedom to engage in deeper conversations regarding personal faith, spirituality and prayer.

Acquaintances who knew my background encouraged me to consider parish nursing—a movement beginning in the United States when Pastor Westberg (1990) realized the potential for nurses to be "ministers of health" in congregations. Canadian nurses, including Lynda Miller (1997) and Joanne Olson (Clarke & Olson, 2000) have implemented educational programs for parish nurses in Canada. Learning more about the relationship between faith and health, I discovered research reporting that people with a strong religious faith are in fact healthier; have stronger immune systems, stronger sense of well-being and life satisfaction and longer lives (Koenig, 1999).

After leaving the health care workforce in 2000, I explored possibilities for parish nursing in my community and volunteered for a parish nurse demonstration project in the local Anglican parish. Visiting as a professional nurse and representative of the church offered opportunities to pray and talk about spiritual matters with parishioners. Parishioners seemed to think they were expected to talk only about health problems, but with gentle encouragement, conversations shifted to other matters close to their hearts and many times they also ministered to me.

Choosing the nursing path

I liken my own spiritual journey through nursing to walking the labyrinth. This ancient practice, healing and integrating mind, body and soul, is now being recovered (West, 2000). Walking the rocky path, circling back and forth towards and away from the centre of the labyrinth, grounds me in my spirituality. Eagerly rushing around each corner, I pause at the core to breathe in fresh air that fills and renews my spirit for the next steps of the passage. Leaves rustle as the wind wisps through the trees; machines rumble in the distance and a robin's chirps welcome me as I emerge from the centre into the outside world.

This spiritual practice is symbolic of the journey to the depths of one's soul. As the circuitous route nears the centre, it veers away to make yet another circuit. For me, it is intertwined with a career path branching in many directions but remaining connected to the source of inspiration for the journey.

I grew up on a farm with a loving family and spiritually grounded in the Moravian[x] church that emphasizes service to others and has a long history of world mission. My life was relatively simple before beginning nursing school so I was unprepared and surprised by the pain and affliction greeting me when entering that path. Caring for young adults in iron lungs and persons of all ages with debilitating and painful illnesses, I asked, "How can a loving God allow people to suffer?" After sharing these questions with my sister, she prayerfully sent me a booklet with "sentences for testing times" as wisdom for the journey:

> *Your guide will keep to no beaten path. He will lead you by a way such as you never dreamed your eyes would look upon. It is your business to learn to be peaceful and safe in God in every situation.*
>
> *To take you to His end by the way you know would profit you little. He chooses for you a way you know not, that you may be compelled into a thousand encounters with Himself which will make the journey memorable to Him and to you.*

Perhaps my purpose was to be a channel of God's love, care for and learn from people in distress in places I never imagined. As my passion for nursing grew, the call and desire to nurse in the North after graduation led me out of the country to Alaska. I thrived in the open spaces of the northern landscape, the warmth of its people and challenges of nursing in a northern hospital before returning to Canada to study public health and outpost nursing. Empathizing with the birth pains of moms in labour, I experienced both the burden of being a pioneer and the ultimate satisfaction of helping give birth to a new program in Outpost Nursing.

Another turn led me back to Alberta to be closer to family. Three years later, my mother died. Our relationship had been strained when I struggled for my independence and freedom to be myself while she realized that my destiny was "different from other girls." A devout woman of faith who prayed and cared deeply for her family, Mom gave us all her blessing as we surrounded her on her death-bed. I cherished that blessing as my grieving soul healed.

Surgery for blockage of the aqueduct in my brain the following year forced me to again pause in the centre to take stock of my life. Having been validated for my rational and academic abilities in the past, I became more conscious of my feminine, intuitive sensibilities. When the shunt blocked two years later while at a nursing conference in Japan, I was comatose until emergency surgery was performed. I later summed up the experience:

> As someone who lost touch with but then regained contact with reality, I know how much I depended on those around me to understand, care and once I regained consciousness, to allow me to recover my independence and self-confidence. I no longer ask "why" all this happened but rather "what am I going to do because it happened?" (Schattschneider, 1978, p.43).

Searching for the centre

In my mid-thirties, as career and church work took over my life, I became physically and spiritually exhausted. My restlessness and constant activity provided an escape from loneliness—part of the human condition which once embraced, led me to a deeper spiritual awareness. When I learned that the Moravian church in Jamaica was asking for help to set up a clinic in downtown Kingston, I offered my assistance. Another time, I visited a rural clinic in Ahuas, a Miskito Indian community on the Honduran east coast. Both undertakings were on behalf of the Moravian Church and wonderful opportunities to apply my nursing knowledge, not as an expert, but as partner and learner. As a result, I was blessed with new perspectives on nursing and life in general.

On my return from Jamaica, I entered a pastoral care education program hoping that it might set a new direction for my career. The demands of management positions had worn me down and I was looking for ways to more openly address the spiritual needs of nurses, including myself, and the people we served. After listening to the fears and anxieties of war veterans in the Veterans' Home, I wrote:

> Do I see or hear the inner yearnings for someone who will listen and care, for freedom from pain and bitterness that becomes heavier with each day, for hope and peace in a life that seems meaningless? These questions are answered when I am open to the flow of life and love that comes from God.

I think of the man with chronic pain. I give him
pills but they don't seem to help. He talks about it so
often. It's hard to listen but when I stop long enough,
I hear him saying, "I'm lonely. I'm depressed. I have
nothing to live for." Can I be with him in all of his
pain? (Schattschneider, 1983, p.3)

Sharing in the profound and sacred moments of
people's lives was indeed "walking on holy ground."
In addition to pastoral care for patients, similar support is needed for nurses dealing with clinical ethical situations and health care politics. Noting the
prevalence of moral distress among nurses, I began
studies in theology with a focus on health care ethics. Recognizing my need for healing, my advisors
encouraged me to balance academic work with sen-
sate activities such as making pottery, walking in the
woods and paying attention to the sounds, smells,
colors and feel of nature. I longed for rest and thirsted
for time by "still waters" to listen and experience
God's Spirit in the silence. Time apart to return to the
centre for reflection to care for my soul was necessary
for the task set before me.

In my thesis work on power relationships in health
care, I asked questions about the forces standing in
the way of humane treatment and balance of power
in health care relationships. Naming the powers was
dangerous work and made me vulnerable to backlash. I learned to recognize the culture or inner spirit
that shapes an organization's attitudes and dynam-
ics. These new insights and questions were not easily

understood or welcomed by the powers that controlled the study and discipline of health care ethics. Curious about my passion for ethics, some were seemingly unable to appreciate my commitment and sense of call to do this work. That calling involved a struggle between the spiritual forces within my own soul and the political and inner forces of organizations. I resented being shut out from possibilities for collaboration but, naively perhaps, continued to call attention to the imbalance of power in the system.

Ethical reflection is a spiritual discipline—definitely work of the soul (Schattschneider, 1992). That reality was validated when an American nurse ethicist, whose writing caught my attention because of its spiritual consciousness, described her work; "I sit at the computer and bleed!" I began to understand that struggle and even suffering is part of the journey when patience, endurance and faith are stretched and tested. Reminding me that this work was more about planting seeds than building empires, mentors and friends affirmed and encouraged me to remain on the path set before me.

My personal life changed dramatically after my move to British Columbia when Lloyd, my husband-to-be, came into my life and reminded me to laugh and not take myself so seriously. We were married on my 53rd birthday! What a blessing to be in relationship with a man who loves and knows me well enough to mirror my heart's desires! But then, there was another twist in the path ahead.

Healing of the soul cut to the core

During the days, months and years following my brother's murder in 1999, as the shock and numbness began to wear off, my path to healing led me again to the centre while I grieved, remembered and gave thanks for my brother's life and the good times we shared. I wrote a journal addressed to him, sharing as we did when he was alive. I knew Doug's spirit was with me as I set out to tell his story, research and document the events leading to his death. The subsequent trial that became a forum for more attacks on the victim cut to the core and soul of our entire family.

This journey could not be easily explained or understood. Entering another wilderness experience and in search for light and meaning in the darkness, I was given a new mission to appeal for reforms to prevent similar events in the future. Some people suggest that crime victims should simply forgive and move on; but that would mean ignoring the pain, trauma and opportunity to make a difference. My request for answers from the offender have gone unanswered but I continue to pray that God will forgive him, dispel his anger and heal his and all spirits broken as a result of my brother's terrible death.

My family was given grace and held together by a strong spiritual core represented by our father who was 88 years of age at the time of his son's death. Dad talked often of his relief that Mom had been spared the horror and pain of their son's murder and frequently expressed his gratitude; "Your mother gave me a wonderful family!" As his health began to fail, he looked forward to joining Mom and others who had already joined the company of saints.

Remembering and honouring elders

Perhaps because we are now elders ourselves, my sister, Mary, and I often talk about our family and elders in our lives. A role model who prepared me for the changes in my body as I approached adolescence, Mary married and moved to a nearby farm where she and her husband raised four children. We took different paths in life but remain connected, and especially appreciate that bond when grieving the deaths of our grandparents, parents and brother and celebrating family rites of passage.

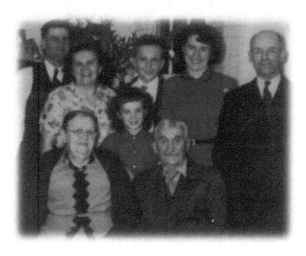

Family Christmas, 1953

I have been gifted with strong and courageous women in my life and even though they preferred not to dwell on their hardships, I wish I knew more of their stories. The adjustments to life in a new country, bearing and raising children, working in the fields and preserving food for the winter naturally kept them in touch with life's ruggedness. Paradoxically, that earthiness was evident by the gentle touch of Mom's hands roughened by her labour of love.

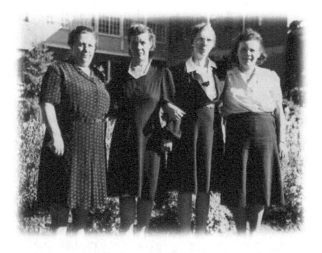

Four sisters: Olga from Chicago, Tillie, Kate, Sophie (Mom) from Edmonton area in 1950

In 1926, at 13 years of age, my mother emigrated with an older sister, Kate, from Poland to Canada. She lived with a farm family and went to school for a few years before moving to the city to work as a housekeeper. In 1934, she married my Dad, a farmer, and together they raised a family; two girls and a boy. I am the youngest.

Conceived and born during the Second World War, as a toddler in my crib, I remember whisperings from the kitchen and warnings in my dreams, "The Russians are coming. The Russians are coming!" During the war, Mom had no contact with her Polish family but when the war ended, she learned that both her parents died in 1943, the year of my birth. For years, a photo of my Polish German grandmother sitting up in bed hung in my parent's bedroom. I often looked into her sad eyes and wondered what she was thinking. After giving birth to 16 children, three who died as infants and two as children, saying farewell to five children emigrating to North America and one going to war, she had reason to be weary and down-hearted!

Only now in my seventieth year can I appreciate the burden she bore and the gift of life she gave my mother and family. The 2010 remembrance of the Russian invasion of Poland provided meaning and context for my childhood dream, my grandmother's sadness and my mother's wish that I stay close to home. Five years before my brother's death, he traveled to Poland to visit our Aunt Alice, Mom's youngest sister, and caught a glimpse of their early lives. Doug spoke often of that pilgrimage.

My paternal grandmother was born in Germany and when 15 years old, immigrated to Canada with an older sister to join a brother who had preceded them. Grandma went to school for a short time to learn English before working as a housekeeper. She married my grandfather who had emigrated with his parents and siblings from Wisconsin to farm in Alberta. Grandma gave birth to two girls and two boys, the youngest being my father. Sadly, both girls died before their first birthday. Dad once said that was why Grandma treasured her grandchildren so much. Our grandparents lived nearby on the neighbouring farm so one of my favorite pastimes as a child was to walk across the field to Grandma and Grandpa's house.

Comparing and celebrating our journeys

One of life's spiritual tasks is to integrate and discover the meaning of personal losses and joys. We celebrate significant milestones, accomplishments in education, work and harvest but when tragedy hits, the pain may seem unbearable. Healing the soul requires time —time not always available to those struggling for survival and elusive when we are tempted to rush the process. I am blessed with time in my senior years to reflect on the journey and cherish precious moments and relationships that have nurtured the core of my being.

I realized at an early age that I was not likely to follow my elders' paths as farm women but will be forever grateful for their example imbedded in my own journey. I have not borne or raised children nor experienced the loss of children as my grandmothers did, but the mothering metaphor describing nursing fits for me. My greatest joy and greatest burden, nursing has given my life meaning and purpose. Honoured to walk with others on sacred paths, I am grateful for mercy and compassion—gifts of God's healing Spirit that guide and sustain us along the way.

When I walk the labyrinth again, the rain falls gently and blesses the journey. I pause to give thanks and pray for rest for the souls who have gone before me and grace for those still walking our paths on earth.

Questions for reflection and discussion

1. What is your understanding of spirituality? Of spiritual needs?
2. How is spiritual care part of nursing?
3. How does your own story affect who you are? Your treatment of other people? Your responses to crisis situations?

TRIBUTE TO FAMILY AND FRIENDS

Throughout my life as a "single career woman", I was blessed with supportive people. Admittedly, there were times of isolation and loneliness but even in those times, people came into my life. Some are life-long childhood or nursing school friends. Others, often nurses, became friends for a particular time and place in a workplace, educational program or faith community. We may have lost contact over the years, but for all of these mentors and friends, I give thanks. In many ways, I am an independent spirit but not so independent that I can live and work without friends and colleagues who I can trust.

As many folk have passed through my life, my family has been a constant source of unconditional love and support. My parents practiced their faith that called for integrity, generosity, concern for family and others in need. My brother, sister and their families provided safe havens and respite when the journey wore me down. Their children and now in turn the next generation of nieces and nephews continue to be a source of great joy.

My husband, Lloyd, joined me during the latest part of the journey and with him, came a new family. Now, not so alone and independent, life has a new dimension!

Thank you to each of you for your gifts of love, friendship and family!

AUTHOR PROFILE

Hazel Joan Schattschneider Magnussen graduated from the University of Alberta Hospital School of Nursing in Edmonton, Alberta in 1964.

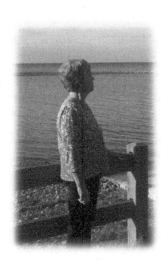

After two years as a staff nurse in an Alaskan Native Hospital, she returned to Canada to continue her studies. In 1969, as the first graduate of the Outpost Nursing Program at Dalhousie University in Halifax, Nova Scotia, she obtained diplomas in Outpost Nursing and Public Health Nursing. Hazel completed her Bachelor of Science degree in nursing at the University of Alberta in 1972.

Hazel worked in management and coordinator positions in public health nursing, programs for the elderly, physically handicapped children and persons with neuromuscular disorders before undertaking studies in health care ethics. After completing a Master of Theological Studies degree from St. Stephen's Theological College in Edmonton, Alberta in 1988, she continued to advocate, consult and write about matters pertaining to health care ethics while employed in short-term positions in nursing education and mental health nursing. Her last nursing position was as community mental health nurse in a program for seniors. Hazel's nursing work and studies took her to five provinces and two territories in Canada, and one American state.

Hazel left the nursing workforce in 2000, a year after the murder of her brother, Dr. Douglas G. Snider, a family physician in northern Alberta. In 2006, she published the book, *A Doctor's Calling: A matter of conscience*, to tell his story. She has advocated for criminal justice reform on behalf of crime victims and change in the medical profession's management of disruptive behaviour by physicians. In 2012, Hazel published the book, *Go North, Young Woman, Go North*, which reviews her northern nursing experience in the 1960's. She maintains an active interest in developments in health care, changes in the nursing profession and the well-being of nurses. Hazel and her husband, Lloyd, live on the west coast of Canada in Parksville, British Columbia.

You can reach Hazel at:

556 Hampstead St.
Parksville, BC V9P 2T7
Ph. 250 586 2036
hazelmag@shaw.ca
www.hazelmagnussen.com

REFERENCES

Arnold, L. (1990). Codependency: Part II: The hospital as a dysfunctional family. *AORN Journal, 51*(6), 1581-1584.

Association of Registered Nurses of BC. (2013). Issue Statement: Staff mix decision-making and nursing practice. Retrieved 7/04/2013 from: http://www.arnbc.ca/images/ pdfs/news-arnbc/ARNBC-Staff-Mix-Statement-June-25.pdf

Austin, W., Goble, E., Leir, B., & Byrne, P. (2009). Compassion Fatigue: The experience of nurses. *Ethics and Social Welfare, 3*(2), 95-214.

Baylis, F., Downie, J., Freedman, B., Hoffmaster, B., Sherwin, S. (1995). *Heath Care Ethics in Canada.* Toronto: Harcourt Brace.

Beagan, B. & Ells, C. (2007). Values that matter, barriers that interfere: The struggle of Canadian nurses to enact their values. *Canadian Journal of Nursing Research,* (4), 37-57.

Beattie, M. (1987). *Codependent No More: How to stop controlling others and start caring for yourself.* San Francisco: Harper & Row.

Benner, P. (1984). *From Novice to Expert: Excellence and power in clinical nursing practice.* Menlo Park California: Addison-Wesley.

Benner, P. & Cook, T. (2011). The spiritual, the ethical and caring. University of California, San Francisco. Retrieved 3/01/2012 from: http://nurseweb.ucsf.edu/public/shobe/ jointstatement.html

Bergen, E., & Fischer, P. (2003). When working hurts. *Nursing BC, 35*(5), 12-15.

Bjorklund, P. (2004). Invisibility, moral knowledge and nursing work in the writings of Joan Liaschenko and Patricia Rodney. *Nursing Ethics, 11*(2), 112-121.

Blum, L. (1991). Moral perception and particularity. *Ethics,* 101 (4), 701-725.

Bradley. Louise. (2010). Commentary: Opening up about mental illness. *Canadian Nurse,* 106 (8), 10.

British Columbia Nurse Practitioner Association. (2012). Minister announces funding so that NPs can be seen in BC, Press Release, May 31, 2012. Retrieved 8/05/2012 from www. bcnpa.org

British Columbia Nurses Union. (2012). Position Statement on Nursing Workload and Patient Safety. Retrieved 1/03/2013 from: https://www.bcnu.org/AboutBCNU/position-stmt-nursing-patient-safety.pdf

British Columbia Nurses' Union. (2013a). VIHA's "Care Delivery Model Redesign" reinventing the 1990's wheel, *Update Magazine,* 32(3), 3. Retrieved 29/10/2013 from: https://www. bcnu.org/news/magazines/2013/update_July-Aug_2013_ web.pdf

British Columbia Nurses Union. (2013b). Protecting ourselves while caring for others. Retrieved 9/09/2013 from: https:// www.bcnu.org/healthsafety/healthsafetybrochure.pdf

British Columbia Nurses Union. (2013c). Professional Practice: Defending and Enhancing Your Practice. Retrieved 8/20/2013 from: https://www.bcnu.org/ ProfessionalPractice/ProfessionalPractice.asp x?page=Licensing%20Education%20Advocacy%20%26%20 Practice% 20(LEAP):search:Leap

Brown, A. (1993). A conceptual clarification of respect. *Journal of Advanced Nursing.* 18 (2), 211-217.

Brown, H. & Rodney, P. (2007). Beyond case studies: Creating capacities for ethical knowledge through story and narrative, In Young. L. & Paterson, L. (Eds), *Teaching Nursing: Developing a Student Centered Learning Environment,* (pp. 141-163). Philadelphia: Lippincott Williams and Wilkins.

Bruce, A., McDonald, C. & McIntyre, M. (2006). Opening the conversation: Dilemmas and possibilities of spirituality and spiritual care In *Realities of Canadian Nursing* edited by M. McIntyre, E. Tomlinson & C. McDonald, (2nd Ed; p. 434-448). Philadelphia: Wolters Kluwer, Lippincott Williams & Wilkins.

Bully Free BC (2012). http://bullyfreebc.ca/legislation.html

Buresh, B. & Gordon, S. (2000). *From Silence to Voice: What nurses know and must communicate to the public*. Ottawa: Canadian Nurses Association.

Cameron, M. (1986). The moral and ethical component of nurse-burnout, *Nursing Management*, Critical Care Management Edition, April p.42B-42E.

Campbell, M.L. & Rankin, J.M. (2006). *Managing to Nurse: Inside Canada's Health Care Reform*. University of Toronto Press.

Canada Safety Council. (2004). Targeting Workplace Bullies. Retrieved 8/20/2004 from www.safety-council.org

Canadian Association of Midwives (2013). Letter to the Editor, *The Globe and Mail*, Retrieved 8/24/2013 from: http://www.canadianmidwives.org/62-news/July-12-2013-CAM-ACSF-Letter-to-the-Editor-The-Globe-and-Mail.html

Canadian Broadcasting Corporation news (2006, Dec 11). Nurses report high levels of abuse, stress. Retrieved 7/27/2011 from: www.cbc,ca/news/canada/story/2006/12/11/nurses-survey.html

CBC (2013, April 13). Nearly 25% of Canadian nurses wouldn't recommend their hospital. Retrieved 05/09/2013 from: http://www.cbc.ca/news/health/story/2013/04/05/hospitals-nurses-survey.html

Canadian Centre for Occupational Health and Safety. (2009). *Violence in the Workplace Prevention* Guide. http://www.ccohs.ca/products/publications/violence.html

Canadian Federation of Nurses Unions (2012). Nursing Workload and Patient Care: Understanding the value of nurses, the effects of excessive workload, and now nurse-patient ratios and dynamic staffing models can help. Retrieved 3/20/2013 from http://www.nursesunions.ca/report-study/nursing-workload-and-patient-care

Canadian Medical Association. (2003). CMA launches centre for physician health and well-being. Retrieved 2/27/12 from: http://www.cma.ca/index.php?ci_id=25562&la_id=1

Canadian Mental Health Association (2013), Depression in the workplace. Retrieved 8/8/2013 from: http://www.cmha.ca/mental_health/depression-in-the-workplace/ Seasonal Affective Disorder. Retrieved 8/08/2013 from: http://www.cmha.ca/mental-health/understanding-mental-illness/mood-disorders/seasonal-affective-disorder/

Canadian Nurse (2010, October). Fatigue: Stories from the frontlines, *Canadian Nurse*, (106 (8), 24-28.

Canadian Nurses Association. (2008). Code of Ethics for Registered Nurses, author. Retrieved 9/01/2012 from: http://www.cna-aiic.ca/~/media/cna/files/en/codeofethics.pdf

Canadian Nurses Association. (2009 a). Position Statement: The Nurse Practitioner. Retrieved 2/22/2013 from: http://www2.cnaaiic.ca/cna/documents/pdf/publications/ps_nurse_ practitioner_e.pdf

Canadian Nurses Association. (2009 b). The Value of Nurses, Fact Sheet. Retrieved 1/03/2013 from: http://www2.cnaaiic.ca/CNA/documents/pdf/publications/ROI_Val ue_Of_Nurses_FS_e.pdf

Canadian Nurses Association. (2009 c). The Next Decade: CNA's vision for nursing and health. Retrieved 9/01/2012 from http://www.cna-aiic.ca/en/on-the-issues/the-next-decade/

Canadian Nurses Association. (2010). Taking action on nurse fatigue. Retrieved 2/27/2013 from: http://www2.cnaaiic. ca/CNA/documents/pdf/publications/PS112_Nu rse_ Fatigue_2010_e.pdf

Canadian Nurses Association. (2011). *Canadian Nurses Association says 'it's about time.* Retrieved 2/22/2013 from: http://www.bcnpa.org/_tiny_mce/plugins/filemanager/ files/CNA_N P_Campaign_Launch.pdf

Canadian Nurses Association (2012a). *A nursing call to action: The health of our nation, the future of our health care system.* Ottawa, ONT: Retrieved 8/27/2012 from: http:// www.cna-aiic.ca/en/canadas-nurses-action-change-with-a- new-blueprint-for-health-care-transformation/

Canadian Nurses Association. (2012b). Nurse Fatigue, Fact Sheet. Retrieved 2/27/2013 from: http://www2.cnaaiic.ca/ CNA/documents/pdf/publications/Fact_She et_Nurse_ Fatigue_2012_e.pdf

Canadian Nurses Association. (2013). Patient plays a greater role in the Fifth Estate series than in the health system. Retrieved 5/09/2013 from: http://www.cna-aiic.ca/en/ patient-plays-greater-role-in-the-fifth-estate-series-than- in-the-health-system/

Canadian Press. (2007). Almost one in five violent incidents occurs in workplace, study finds. Retrieved 2/18/2007 from: www.macleans.ca/article.jsp?content=n021602A

Cauthorne-lindstrom, C. & Hrabe, D. (1990). Co-dependent behaviors in managers: A script for failure, *Nursing Management,* 21(2), 34-39.

Centre for Applied Research in Mental Health and Addiction (CARMHA) (2012). *Guarding Minds at Work; Workplace guide to psychological health and safety.* Retrieved 8/06/2013 from: http://www.guardingmindsatwork.ca/info

Cheperdak, D. & Sudbury, F. (2011). Nurse practitioner an asset for care home. *Times Colonist,* Nov. 17, A11.

Clarke, C. (2010). Why civility matters, *Reflections on nursing leadership 36(1)*. Retrieved 2/7/2011 from: http://www. reflectionsonnursingleadership.org/Pages/Vol36_1_Clark2_civility.aspx

Clarke, M.B. & Olson, J.K. (2000). *Nursing within a faith community: Promoting health in times of transition.* Thousand Oaks: Sage.

College of Physicians and Surgeons of Alberta. (2010). Managing Disruptive Behavior in the Healthcare Workplace. Retrieved 10/12/2011 from: http://www.cpsa.ab.ca/Libraries/Res/MDB_guidance_document_to olkit_for_web.pdf

College of Registered Nurses of British Columbia (2013). What Nurses Do. Retrieved 3/23/2013 from: https://crnbc.ca/WhatNursesDo/Pages/Default.aspx

Coloroso, B. (2002). *The bully, the bullied and the bystander.* Toronto: Harper Collins.

Curtin, L. & Flaherty, J. (1982). *Nursing ethics: Theories and pragmatics.* Bowie, Maryland: Robert J. Brady.

Dellasega, C. (2005). *Mean girls grown up; Adult women who are still queen bees, middle bees and afraid to bees. New Jersey:* John Wiley.

Dellasega, C. (2009). Bullying among nurses, *American Journal of Nursing,* 109(1), 52-58.

Dellasega, C. (2011). *When nurses hurt nurses: Recognizing and overcoming the cycle of bullying.* Honor Society of Nursing, Sigma Theta Tau International.

Dickinson, Gordon T. (1966 October). Editorial from Canadian *Medical Association Journal* 94:552 reprinted in *Among the Deep Sea Fishers,* p. 66-69.

Doucet, H. (1984 Spring). New approaches to death: Ethics and palliative Care. *CHAC Review,* pp.15-18.

Downie, J. (2013, Oct 21). The Supreme Court decision in Rasouli, IMPACT ETHICS. Retrieved 26/10/2013 from: http://impactethics.ca/2013/10/21/the-supreme-court-decision-in-rasouli/

Duncan, S., Hyndman, K., Estabrooks, C., Hesketh, K., Humphrey, C., Wong, S. (2001). Nurses' experience of violence in Alberta and British Columbia hospitals. *Canadian Journal of Nursing Research, 32(4),* 57-78.

Edelwich, J. with Brodsky, A. (1980). *Burn-out: Stages of disillusionment in the helping professions.* Rocky Hill, CT: Human Sciences Press.

Ferguson-Pare, M. (2008, January/February). The gift of respect, *Registered Nurse Journal,* RNAO, p. 5.

Frank, A.W. (2005). *The Renewal of Generosity: Illness, medicine and how to live.* Chicago: University of Chicago Press.

Freedman, B. (1981). A prolegomenon to the allocation of responsibility in hierarchical organization: nurses and physicians. In M. Staum & D. Larsen (Eds), *Doctors, Patients and Society: Power and Authority in Medical Care. Waterloo, On:* Wilfred Laurier.

Glendel, H. (2000). Disruptive Behaviors, Personality Problems, and Boundary Violations. In H. Goldman, M. Myers & L. Dickstein (Eds.), *Handbook of Physician Health.* American Medical Association.

Globe & Mail Editorial. (2012). Between medicine and morals, *The Globe and Mail,* December 11, A12.

Gordon, S. (Ed). (2010). *When chicken soup isn't enough: Stories of nurses standing up for themselves, their patients and their profession.* Ithaca: Cornell University Press.

Great Place to Work Institute. (2012). www.greatplacetowork.ca/our-approach/what-is-a-great-workplace

Growe, S.J. (1991). *Who Cares: The crisis in Canadian nursing.* Toronto: McClelland and Stewart.

Haines, J. (1997). Questions from an Inquest. *Canadian Nurse,* 93(10), 3.

Hamric, A. B. (2010). Moral distress and nurse-physician relationships. *Virtual Mentor,* 12 (1), 6-11. Retrieved 2/28/2013 from: http://virtualmentor.ama-assn.org/2010/01/ ccas1-1001.html

Handbury, E. (1975). *NURSE.* Toronto: McClelland & Stewart.

Hardingham, L. (2004). Integrity and moral residue: nurses as participants in a moral community. *Nursing Philosophy,* 5, 127-134.

Hardingham, L. (2006). Ethical and legal Issues in nursing. In M. McIntyre & C. McDonald (Eds.), *Realities of Canadian Nursing,* (2nd Ed; pp. 327-333.) Toronto: Lippincott.

Harrision, B. (1981). The power of anger in the work of love. *Union Seminary Quarterly Review* XXXVI (Supplementary), 41-57.

Health Canada. (2006). Nursing issues: Primary health care nurse practitioners. Retrieved 2/22/2013 from: http://www. hc-sc.gc.ca/hcs-sss/pubs/nurs-infirm/onp-bpsi-fs-if/2006-np-ip-eng.php.

Henderson, A. (2010). Nurses' experiences of workplace violence: Toward effective intervention. Final Report. Workplace BC Focus on Tomorrow 2006 Competition. Retrieved 12/28/2011 from: http://www.worksafebc.com/ contact_us/research/funding_decision s/assets/pdf/2006/ RS2006_OG17.pdf

Herr, J. (1976). Psychology of aging: An overview. In Irene Mortensen Burnside (Ed.), *Nursing and the aged.* (pp. 36-44). New York: McGraw Hill.

Hesketh, K., Duncan, S., Estabrooks, C., Reimer, M., Giovannetti, P., Hyndman, Acorn, S. (2003). Workplace violence in Alberta and British Columbia hospitals. *Health Policy*, 63, 311-321.

Houshmand, M., O'Reilly, J., Robinson, S. & Wolff, A. (2012). Escaping bullying: The simultaneous impact of individual and unit-level bullying on turnover intentions. *Human Relations*, 65(7), 901-918.

Hutchinson M, Jackson, D, Vickers M and Wilkes L. (2006). Workplace bullying in nursing: towards a more critical organizational perspective. *Nursing Inquiry*, 13(2), 118-126.

Jameton, A. (1984). *Nursing Practice: the ethical issues*. Englewood Cliffs, NJ: Prentice Hall.

Joffe, A.R. (2011). Why is there concern about organ donation after cardiac death? *Health Care Ethics Today*, 19 (1), 3-5. Retrieved 12/01/2011 from: http://www.bioethics.ualberta. ca/en/~/media/dossetor/Health%20E thics%20Today/ HET%20Vol%2019%20No1%202011.pdf

Kaufert, J. & O'Neil, J. (1990). Biomedical rituals and informed consent: Native Canadians and the negotiation of clinical trust. In G. Weisz (Ed.), *Social Science Perspectives on Medical Ethics*. (pp.42-63), The Netherlands: Kluwer Academic Press.

Koenig, Harold G. (1999). *The Healing Power of Faith: Science explores medicine's last frontier*. New York: Simon and Schuster.

Laschinger, H. , Leiter, M., Day, A., & Gilen, D. (2009). Workplace empowerment, incivility and burnout: impact on staff nurse recruitment and retention outcomes. *Journal of Nursing Management*, 1, 302-311.

Leininger, M. (1990). Culture: The conspicuous missing link to understand ethical and moral dimensions of human care. In M. Leininger (Ed.), *Ethical and moral dimensions of care*. Detroit: Wayne State Univ.

Lindh, I., Severinsson, E. & Berg, A. (2007). Moral Responsibility: A relational way of being. *Nursing Ethics,* 14(2), 129-139.

Magnussen, H. (2003, Sept 1). "After Violence Strikes", Over to You Page. *MACLEAN'S,* p.46.

Magnussen, H. (2006). *A Doctor's Calling: A matter of conscience.* Parksville, B.C.: Wembley.

Mann, K., Gordon, J., & MacLeod, A. (2009). Reflection and reflective practice in health professions education: a systemic review. *Advances in Health Science Education,* 14, 595-621.

Marriner-Tomey, A. (1989). *Nursing Theorists and their work.* Toronto: Mosby.

Mental Health Commission of Canada (2012, April 27). Media Release: Mental Health Commission of Canada introduces new guide to enhance workplace mental health. Retrieved 4/27/212 from: www.mentalhealthcommission.ca

Mental Health Commission of Canada (2013, January 16). Media Release: National Standard of Canada for psychological health and safety in the workplace released. *Retrieved 6/22/2013 from:* http://www. mentalhealthcommission.ca/English/node/4089

Miller, L.W. (Winter, 1997) Nursing though the lens of faith: A conceptual model. *Journal of Christian Nursing,* 14(1), 17-23.

Mitchell, G. & Santopinto, M. (1988). An alternative to nursing diagnosis. *Canadian Nurse, 84 (10),* 25-28.

Molzahn, A.E., & Shields, L. (2008). Why is it so hard to talk about spirituality? *Canadian Nurse,* (104 (1), 25-29.

Mooney, N. (2005). *I can't believe she did that: Why women betray other women at work,* New York: St.Martin's Griffin.

Nanaimo Daily News Editorial (2000). "Wake up to nursing shortages," *Nanaimo Daily News,* Jan. 21, p. A8.

National Aboriginal Council of Midwives (2013). NACM Mission and Vision. Retrieved 8/24/2013 from: http://aboriginalmidwives.ca/about

Nightingale, Florence (1914). A selection from Miss Nightingale's addresses to probationers and nurses of the Nightingale School of St. Thomas Hospital. London: Macmillan & Co. Retrieved 3/31/2013 from: http://archive.org/stream/florencenightingoonighiala/florencenighti ngoonighiala_djvu.txt

O'Neil, J. (1989). The cultural and political context of patient dissatisfaction in cross-cultural clinical encounters: A Canadian Inuit study. *Medical Anthropology, 3*(4), 325-44.

Ontario Ministry of Health and Long Term Care. (2013). Nurse Practitioner led clinics. Retrieved 2/22/2013 from: http://health.gov.on.ca/transformation/np_clinics/np_mn.html

Ontario Nurses Association. (2012). New nurse health program planning, Highlights—June Provincial Coordinators' Meeting, p. 2-3. Retrieved 2/28/2013 from: www.ona.org'documents/file/onanews/ona_June12highlights.

Parse, R. (1992). Human Becoming: Parse's theory of nursing, *Nursing Science Quarterly, 5*(1), 35-42.

Picard, A. (2000*). Critical Care: Canadian nurses speak for change,* Toronto: Harper Collins. (A Phyllis Bruce Book)

Picard, A. (2012). Nurse practitioners: an untapped resource, *The Globe and Mail, Jan. 17, L6.*

Picard, A. (2013). Midwives: Underused and misused assets in Canada, *The Globe and Mail, July 10.* Retrieved 8/24/2013 from: http://www.theglobeandmail.com/life/health-and-fitness/health/midwives-underused-and-misused-assets/article13133123

Puddester, D. (2008) Honouring the Dead, *CMAJ, 179*(1), 57-58. http://www.cmaj.ca/content/179/1/57.full.pdf+html

Quinn, C., & Smith, M. (1987). *The Professional Commitment: Issues and ethics in nursing,* Toronto: Saunders.

Rachlis, M. (2004). *Prescription for excellence: How innovation is saving Canada's heath care system,* First edition, Toronto: Harper Collins.

Randle, J. (2003). Bullying in the nursing profession. *Journal of Advanced Nursing,* 43(4), 395-401.

Randle, J., Stevenson, K., & Grayling, I. (2007). Reducing workplace bullying in healthcare organizations. *Nursing Standard,* 21(22), 49-56.

Rankin, N. (1988). I see and am silent. *Canadian Critical Care Nursing Journal,* 5(2), 6-7.

Registered Nurses Association of British Columbia. (2001 December). A question of values. *Nursing BC,* p.13.

Registered Nurses Association of Ontario. (1987). RNAO Responds: A nursing perspective on events at the Hospital of Sick Children and the Grange Inquiry. Toronto: RNAO.

Rest, J. (1982). A psychologist looks at the teaching of ethics. The *Hastings Center Report,* 2(1), 29-36.

Roach, M. S.M. (1992). *The human act of caring: A blueprint for the health professions,* Ottawa: Canadian Hospital Association, Ottawa.

Rocker, C. (2008). Addressing nurse to nurse bullying to promote nurse retention, *The Online Journal of Issues in Nursing,* 13(3), Retrieved 4/31/ 2013 from: http://www.nursingworld.org/MainMenuCategories/ANAMarketpla ce/ANAPeriodicals/OJIN/TableofContents/vol132008/ No3Sept08/Ar ticlePreviousTopic/NursetoNurseBullying. html

Rocker, C. (2012). *Fatigue and nurses' perspective of working the night shift: A quantitative study.* (unpublished) Dissertation for completion of Doctor of Health Administration degree from University of Phoenix, Arizona.

Rodney, P. (1988). Moral distress in critical care nursing. *Canadian Critical Care Nursing Journal,* 5(2), 9-11.

Rodney, P., Varcoe, C., Storch, J., McPherson, G., Mahoney, K., Brown, H., Pauly, B., Hartrick, G., & Starzomski, R. (2002). Navigating towards a moral horizon: a multisite qualitative study of ethical practice in nursing. *Canadian Journal of Nursing Research,* 34(3), 75-102.

Rolheiser, R. (1999). *The holy longing: The search for a Christian spirituality,* New York: Random.

Rosenstein, A. (2002). Nurse-Physician relationships: impact on nurse satisfaction and retention. *American Journal of Nursing,* 102(6), 26-34.

Ross-Kerr, J.C. (1998). *Prepared to Care: Nurses and Nursing in Alberta.* Edmonton: University of Alberta Press.

Russell, L. (1983). Human liberation in a feminist perspective, Philadelphia: Westminster.

Ruth-Sahd, L. (2003). Reflective Practice: A critical analysis of data-based studies and implications for nursing education. *Journal of Nursing Education,* 42 (11), 488-495.

Sabo, B. (2011). Reflecting on the concept of compassion fatigue, Posted: 7/08/2011; *OJIN: The Online Journal of Issues in Nursing,* 2011:16(1) American Nurses Association. Retrieved 7/19/2012 from: http://compassionfatigue.ca/wpcontent/uploads/2011/09/Reflecting-on-the-Concept-of-Compassion-Fatigue-printer-friendly.pdf

St. Pierre, I. (2012). The link between organizational justice and nursing workload, *Nursing Workload and Patient Care,* Canadian Federation of Nurses Unions, p 9.

Sankey, D. (2005). Resilience is a vital workplace skill. *Oceanside Star, Jan. 5, B1.*

Schattschneider, H. (1969, Winter). Adventure into outpost nursing. *Dalhousie Medical Review,* p. 57-60.

Schattschneider, H. (1969, January). Outpost Nurse, *Among the Deep Sea Fishers*, p. 117-120.

Schattschneider, H. (1977). Community Resources for the Elderly: Day Hospital. *Canadian Nurse, 73 (4)*, 47-49.

Schattschneider, H. (1978). Arigato, Japan. *Canadian Nurse*, 74 (6), 42-43.

Schattschneider, H. (1983, February). A nurse's reflections, *The Beat*, U of A Hospitals Staff bulletin, p. 2-3.

Schattschneider, H. (1988). Power in physician-nurse –patient relationships: A nursing perspective, Thesis (unpublished) completed for Master of Theological Studies Degree, St. Stephen's Theological College, Edmonton, Alberta.

Schattschneider, H. (1990). Power relationships between physician and nurse. *Humane Medicine, 6* (3), 197-201.

Schattschneider, H. (1991). Transplant ethics need study: Should animal-to human transplants be accepted practice? (Letter to the editor), *Edmonton Journal, Oct. 1, A11*.

Schattschneider, H. (1992). Ethics for the Nineties: Will nurses continue to care? *Canadian Nurse, 88* (10), 16-18.

Schattschneider, H. (1993, June). Advance treatment directives: A nurse ethicist's view. *AARN newsletter*, p.18-19.

Seedhouse, D. (2009). *Ethics: The Heart of Health Care*. Third Edition, UK: Wiley.

Shalof, T. (2008). The Making of a Nurse, Toronto: McClellan Stewart.

Shalof, T. (Ed.) (2009). *Lives in the Balance: Nurses stories from the ICU*. Toronto: Emblem Editions.

Sibbald, B. (1999). RN=Really Neglected, angry nurses say. *Canadian Medical Association Journal*, 160(10), 1490-91. http://www.cmaj.ca/content/160/10/1490.full.pdf+html

Sinclair, C.M. (2000) *Report of the Manitoba pediatric cardiac inquest.* Winnipeg: Manitoba Provincial Court. Retrieved 3/12/2013 from: http://www.pediatriccardiacinquest.mb.ca/pdf/index.html

Sinnema, J. (2011). Nurse practitioners fill 'unique niche. *Edmonton Journal, Oct. 31, A3.*

Spilman, J. (2013, Jan. 17). The Cost of Caring: Compassion Fatigue recovery and resilience, Handout and notes from lecture at Spirit at Work Luncheon, Vancouver, BC.

Storch, J., & Kenny, L. (2007). Shared moral work of nurses and physicians. *Nursing Ethics, 14 (4),* 478-491.

Storch, J., Rodney, P., Pauly, B., Fulton, T., Stevenson, l., Newton, L., Makaroff, K. (2009). Enhancing ethical climates in nursing work environments. *Canadian Nurse,* 105(3), 20-25.

Thomas, J.E. (1988, Fall). Ethics: Nursing at the crossroads, *The RNAO News,* p.29-30.

Travelbee, J. (1966). *Interpersonal Aspects of Nursing.* Philadelphia: F.A. Davis.

Ulrich, B. (1992). *Leadership and Management according to Florence Nightingale,* Connecticut: Appleton & Lange.

University of Alberta. (2013). Educating midwives in Canada's Arctic. Retrieved 8/26/2013 from: http://news.ualberta.ca/newsarticles/2013/may/educating-midwives-in-canadas-arctic

Varcoe, C., Pauly, B., Storch, J., Newton., & Makaroff, K., (2012). Nurses' perception of and responses to morally distressing situations, *Nursing Ethics,* 19(4), 488-500.

Veatch, R.M. (1981). Nursing Ethics, physician ethics and medical ethics. *Law, Medicine and Healthcare,* 9(6), 17-19.

Webster, G.C., & Baylis, F. (2000). Moral Residue. In S.B. Rubin & l. Zoloth (Eds.), *Margin of error: the ethics of mistakes in the practice of medicine*. Hagerstown, MD: University Publishing Group.

West, M.G. (2000). *Exploring the Labyrinth; A guide for healing and spiritual growth*. New York: Broadway.

West, M.L. (2003). *The Shoes of the Fisherman*. New Milford, C.T.: Toby.

Westberg, G.E. (1990). *The Parish Nurse*. Minneapolis: Augsburg.

Westhues, K. (2002). At the Mercy of the Mob, *OHS Canada* 18(80), 30-36. Retrieved 8/18/2010 from: http://www.arts. uwaterloo.ca/~kwesthue/ohs-canada

Wilson, B (1977). *To Teach this Art*. Edmonton: Halamshire.

Wink, W. (1984). *Naming the Powers*. Philadelphia: Fortress.

Wink, W. (1986). *Unmasking the Powers*. Philadelphia: Fortress.

Wink, W. (1993). *Cracking the Gnostic Code*. Atlanta: Scholars.

Winslow, G.R. (1984, June). From loyalty to advocacy: A new metaphor for nursing. *The Hastings Center Report*, 32-40.

WorkSafe BC (2013). Bullying and Harassment Prevention Tool Kit. Retrieved 11/01/2013 from: http://www2.worksafebc. com/Topics/BullyingAndHarassment/Reso urces. asp?reportID=37260

Yarling, R.R. & McElmurry, B.J. (1986).The moral foundation of nursing, *Advances in Nursing Science*, 8(2), 63-73.

Yeo, M., Rodney, P., Khan, P. & Moorhouse, A. (2010 a). Integrity. In YM. Yeo, A. Moorhouse, P. Khan, & P. Rodney (Eds.), *Concepts and Cases in Nursing Ethics*. (3rd Edition, pp.349-387). Canada: Broadview.

Yeo, M., Rodney, P., Moorhouse, A., & Khan, P. (2010 b). Justice. In M. Yeo, A. Moorhouse, P. Khan, & P. Rodney (Eds.), *Concepts and Cases in Nursing Ethics*. (3rd Edition, pp. 293-347). Canada: Broadview.

NOTES:

i   The Colonel Mewburn Pavilion, which opened in
    1946, was named after Dr. Frank Mewburn, WW1
    veteran, professor and director of surgery from
    1921-29. A tunnel connected it to the University of
    Alberta Hospital.

ii   The report of the Royal Commission on Health
    Services (commonly referred to as the Hall
    Commission Report) also laid the foundation for
    a National Medicare system. Federal Medicare
    legislation was passed in December 1966.

iii   Frobisher Bay was renamed Iqaluit in 1987. In
    1999, the eastern part of the Northwest Territories
    became a new territory— Nunavut.

iv   According to minutes of the Dalhousie University
    Senate meeting on March 22, 1999, a proposal for a
    Diploma in Nurse Practitioner Studies for Remote
    and Under-Serviced Communities was approved.
    The proposal was a major modification of the
    dormant Outpost Nursing Program.

v   According to Mosby's Medical Dictionary (2009),
    the term, iatrogenic, refers to consequences
    "caused by treatment or diagnostic procedures. An
    iatrogenic disorder is a condition that is caused by
    medical personnel or procedures" or that develops
    through exposure to the environment of a health
    care facility.

vi   Nursing professor Shannon Spenceley from the University of Lethbridge (2013) will lead a timely research project, funded by the Alzheimer Society, to examine moral distress experienced by staff in care facilities caring for residents with dementia. Retrieved 9/03/3013 from http://www.uleth.ca/notice/display.html?b=300&s=18993

vii   An edition of *Health Care Ethics Today* featured discussion about issues related to death and introduced by its editor, Dr. Paul Byrne (2011). Retrieved 2/23/13 from http://www.bioethics.ualberta.ca/en/~/media/dossetor/Health%20Ethics% 20Today/HET%20Vol%2019%20No1%20 2011.pdf

viii   Jocelyn Downie (2013), professor of medicine and law at Dalhousie University, explains the Supreme Court's ruling in an Ontario case, The Supreme Court decision in Rasouli, IMPACT ETHICS. Retrieved 10/24/2013 from http://impactethics.ca/2013/10/21/the-supreme-court-decision-in-rasouli/

ix   See report on research and discussion of ethical implications of organ donation practices in Kirkey, S. (2013, Oct. 28). "Fewer brain death patients means drop in organ donations, researchers say." *Vancouver Sun*. Retrieved 10/28/2013 from http://www.vancouversun.com/health/Fewer+brain+dead+patients+means+drop+organ+donations/9092412/story.html

x   The Moravian Church is a Protestant denomination founded in 1457 in Czechoslovakia. The Moravian worldwide mission movement began in 1732. See http://www.moravian.ca/docs/mc.html

INDEX

33 (*see also* patients);
power, xi–xii, 43, 45–49,
61–62, 84–85, 106–7,
119; subject of author's
master's thesis, 43–44,
130–31. *See also* bullying;
nurses; physicians;
psychological health and
safety; workplace culture
resilience, 89
respect: aboriginal people,
21; necessary for safe
workplace, 113, 115–16,
117, 119–21; nursing, 119;
nursing ethic, 57; other
team members, 27, 45;
patients, 31–34
Rest, James, 58
resuscitation, prolonging
life, 40–41
Roach, Simone, 123
Rocker, Carol, 96–97, 114
Rodney, Patricia, 46, 60, 80,
83, 90
Rolheiser, Ronald, 123
Ross-Kerr, Janet, 74
Royal Commission on
Health Services, 7, 158

S

Sabo, Brenda, 98
Saskatchewan: nurse
practitioners, 24;
personal harassment,110
Schattschneider, Hazel. *See*
Magnussen, Hazel J.
Seasonal Affective Disorder,
93–94
Seedhouse, David, xv–xvi

seniors: Day Hospital
program, 28–29; health
needs, 84
Serenity Prayer, 91–92
serotonin, 93
"silent power of a consistent
life," 69
Snider, Doug, 49, 111–12, 132,
135
Spenceley, Shannon, 159
Spilman, Jan, 98
spirituality: better health,
125; definition, 123;
ethical reflection,
xv–xvi, 131; grief, 67,
132, 136; inhibited in
science based health
care, 124; life's journey,
136; nursing, 6–7, 47;
questioning God,
127; recovering from
compassion fatigue, 98;
walking the labyrinth,
xviii
St. Anthony, Newfoundland,
17
St. Pierre, Isabelle, 83
St. Stephen's Theological
College, 43
Storch, Janet, 48
stress. *See* burnout;
depression; moral
distress; workload
student nurses: bullying,
107, 112–13; depression
and suicide, 75–76
suicide, nurses, 75, 94
Supreme Court of Canada,
Rasouli decision, 159

X
xenographs, 67–68

Y
Yeo, Michael, 46, 83, 90
Youngson, nurse, 62